The Little Book of Positive Birth Stories

A collection of positive birth stories to support you
throughout your pregnancy and labour.

Claire Fulton

The Little Book of Positive Birth Stories: A collection of positive birth stories to support you throughout your pregnancy and labour.

Claire Fulton

Published 2023
© 2023 Claire Fulton
www.thenurturenest.co.uk

ISBN: 9798852606884

Cover design by Louise Symes

This book offers general information and people's own experiences for interest only and does not consititue or replace individualised professional midwifery or medical care and advice.

Acknowledgements

Thank you to all the incredible, powerful women who have taken the time to write out and share their story in order for me to create this book. Without their input this book could not have been created and I am so grateful.

I dedicate this book to my own two hypnobabies, Elle and Amelie. My experiences being pregnant and giving birth to you both is what started me on this amazing journey.

About the Creator

Claire Fulton is a passionate and experienced hypnobirthing teacher, doula and also a mother of two. She has seen first-hand the power of hypnobirthing and how a positive mindset can change the birth experience for the better. Claire is also the creator and presenter of the number 1 podcast, The Hypnobirthing Podcast, with her aim being to make hypnobirthing as accessible as possible and change the narrative around birth to make it positive, exciting and informed.

Claire knows that the current negative culture and view of childbirth is damaging to those preparing for this milestone event and that if we were inundated with positive stories, positive language and excitement about childbirth, how different we might feel.

All the stories in this book are real stories, written in the words of the person themselves. They are divided up by type of birth, so you can get a sense of how each and every type of birth can be a positive one.

Additional resources available from Claire Fulton
www.thenurturenest.co.uk
Instagram/the_nurture_nest
The Hypnobirthing Podcast

CONTENTS

BREECH..6

CAESAREAN..13

HOME..19

HOSPITAL..46

INDUCTION...73

WATER..102

VBAC..133

BREECH BIRTH

The birth of Chala

Our little one flipped at 37 weeks much to my surprise as my first, Willow, was born vaginally head down, no curve balls thrown, so I hadn't even really thought about breech at all. I was having a prenatal massage when she turned, it was like a jolt going through my body! I was in denial so didn't mention anything when we went to our midwife check-up, the homebirth midwife picked up on it immediately and sent us to the hospital for a scan to confirm. I was very wary of going to the hospital and getting swept up in the system. Sure enough they immediately jumped to heavily suggesting I book an elective caesarean section should the ECV (external cephalic version) be unsuccessful. It was overwhelming and I felt as though something was "wrong" with me. I felt pressured to try an ECV but we went home first and did a lot of research. The internet is amazing. Chris and I decided to try the ECV after meeting with the doctor, who was lovely and gentle and understanding. It was unsuccessful and now we know that the cord was wrapped around Chala's head twice so that could have been what stopped her. I don't know if it was the right thing to try the ECV. I found it to be a very emotional experience, it was also quite painful – more so afterwards than during. So I moved on and decided to embrace it as I was now 38 weeks. I didn't try moxibustion or anything else apart from continuing on with my daily yoga practice (which I did all along anyway). I let go of my homebirth plan because I couldn't find anyone in my area with the experience to support me. I contacted the head of midwifery at the hospital and sent her my VBB plan and request for second birth partner (my doula) which was granted. I also spoke with Kemi Birth Joy Johnson who was just absolutely so supportive and reaffirmed my faith in myself. I filled my mind with positive VBB podcasts and stories and websites and videos. I also wrote an emergency caesarean plan and spent a little bit of time thinking on that.

My waters broke on Friday 22nd October night/Saturday morning at 1:30am. I was 38 weeks and 5 days. I woke up to turn over in bed and as I did there was a "pop" and I jumped up and into the bathroom to see. The waters were red with quite a lot blood which was a bit scary. We called the triage line and after speaking to a midwife I was told to come straight in, the midwife on the phone was so excited when she heard I was planning on a VBB. This was really reassuring. The hospital was over an hour drive away, my Dad drove us, and when we arrived I was still losing quite a lot of blood. I allowed the doctor to do a vaginal examination. I was 3cm. They asked if I wanted to do a caesarean section because they didn't know where the blood was coming from. I declined and asked to wait a little longer as I felt fine and baby was happy. Surges had begun inconsistently. They agreed I could wait but they asked to put a cannula in my hand so they had quick access to a vein should the bleeding get worse very quickly. That was scary and also very uncomfortable. But I agreed as I felt it was a fair compromise. I also agreed to continuous monitoring in the form of wireless doppler. We covered the monitor with a scarf and turned the volume off so it wasn't too intense. It was actually nice because the data is sent to the midwives outside the room and if everything is steady it means they don't need to come in and keep checking.

While I was still bleeding there was a feeling in the air that I would be going to theatre. I didn't want to think about it so I asked Jo (my doula) and Chris if we could get the room ready. They put the fairy lights up, and my birth affirmations and our oils. I used clary sage, Lavender and frankincense.

My labour took a few hours to "establish" because I kept getting interrupted by doctors giving me their unwanted opinions about my decision for a VBB. But the bleeding had stopped and waters were coming through clear now so my worry lessened. I got really annoyed with two male doctors pressuring me to talk about my caesarean section plan should labour fail to establish within their timeframe since waters had broken. It had been only 7 hours since my waters broke (I still had plenty of time even by their protocol of 24hrs) and the bleeding had stopped, plus my surges had started which he didn't bother to ask about. I just ignored them. When they left I asked my doula and partner to go and speak to our midwife. They told her no more people in the room. Only her. No one else. They gave me my safe space back. My doula, Jo, was amazing. Her presence in the room reinforced the respect for my birth plan. She was gentle but encouraged me through the whole way. After a particularly big surge she said "well, you never have to do that one again!" I loved that. I'm not sure whether or not to share this part but its part of the story so I guess I should! I remembered a post I'd seen on Instagram about an orgasm being 22 times more relaxing than the average tranquilizer. I felt I was chasing the waves and they were eluding me because I didn't feel so safe. The surges had gone from 7 minutes apart to inconsistently 30 minutes, 40 minutes, and 20 minutes apart. SO FRUSTRATING. So I decided to try it, I didn't say anything, I just went into the bathroom. Immediately, and I mean immediately, after that my surges came on properly, soon they were just 2-3 minutes apart and lasting at least a minute each wave. I used my hypnobirthing and essential oils on a little paper towel that I could smell during contractions. My doula supported my back beautifully with pressure points. Wherever I was in the room,

Jo would jump over as soon as the wave started and hold my back through it.

Chris was amazing, reassuring and loving and supportive. He said to me "remember this is the last time to feel your baby moving inside you, this is your last birth, enjoy it". This really hit me, he knew how much I was looking forward to the birth. I felt everything. I felt so connected to Chala, I could feel her wiggling her bum as she moved down through my body. I felt so emotional knowing that another soul was joining our family, that Willow would be a big sister. Chris was emotional too, he told me later that it was more emotional this time around because he knew the love he had for Willow and that he would feel this for the baby too. As cheesy as it may sound, he was my protector and my rock. When those male doctors came in, Chris came and stood behind me and put his arms around me wrapping me up and making a barrier between me and them.

After about an hour, the midwife came to check in as she noticed from the monitor that things had ramped up a lot. She asked to do another vaginal examination. I agreed but asked that she didn't tell me my dilation, she was a bit surprised but agreed.

After the birth she told me I was 9cm, but after the check she just said we were going to get ready to meet baby soon. She began to get the room ready and spoke to me about staying standing and trusting my body to guide me into whatever position I needed to be in. I was on my yoga mat, kneeling and leaning into Chris. I began to shake and I knew I was in transition. All I could think was the only way is through this. It was much more intense than Willow's because I didn't have the water to support me. I missed the water so much. My midwife gently guided me in trusting my body and reassured me she would be hands off unless absolutely necessary and would talk to me the whole time. She told me not to push until there was just no way I couldn't.

She told me to breathe and take my time through each contraction. I couldn't disappear completely as I had done in Willow's labour, I had to keep coming back to listen to the midwife's guidance. She was calm and confident and guided me perfectly. I could hear her voice clearly.

Pushing began when I absolutely could not breathe through anymore and lasted just 11 minutes, the midwife called in a second midwife to be present. Jo was filming and taking photos on Chris's phone. This part was hard, I knew we had to do this calmly but efficiently. I knelt on my yoga mat and lent into Chris. Her one foot came out first, then her bum with her other leg. She was hanging beneath me, my midwife said I could reach down and then I felt her! I didn't really understand what part of her I was feeling, it was her bum, so soft and squishy. We discovered we were having another baby girl! I cried! I moved into a standing position. Then the midwife could see her arms were caught over her head. She asked me if she could assist her because she was a little stuck. I agreed, it was very intense but I see in the video how gentle she was releasing the arms. After the arms were out it was a huge relief. Now I could feel the hardness of her head, it was so hard after the squishy body! The midwife said to wait for the next surge and when it came to give it everything. There was a moment of complete peace while Chala was hanging out of me, supported by the midwife who kept reminding me not to sit down as I would sit on my baby! The room was completely quiet apart from my music. The final wave came, I moved into a lunge and then a wide legged "goddess" squat, I gave everything and she was out! The midwife told me to stand still as she unwound the cord from around Chala's neck after which came her first cry as she was passed straight to me.

We did it! Euphoria. Chala was here with us. She was so alert and so perfect.

The placenta took about an hour and the contractions were stronger than I remember from last time but we enjoyed our golden hour, we only cut the cord after 45 minutes. She scored 8/10 on the Apgar Scale at birth and 10/10 after a few minutes. She began rooting and immediately latched on and started asking my body to feed her.

Later I was told that there were doctors and a neonatal specialist outside the door while I was birthing Chala. But the midwife told them she would press the button if she needed help and otherwise to stay outside. She was absolutely incredible. I feel so lucky to have had her assist us in this birth. Chala Nichola Rodgers was born at 12:54pm and weighed 3.4kg and we were discharged a couple of hours later.

No stitches for me this time around. I know it's a bit of a long story but I also know there are others out there looking to stock up on positive VBB stories so this is for you. Our bodies are amazing and however we birth our babies, head down, head up, through a section, we are all incredible.

Hannah and baby Chala

CAESAREAN BIRTH

The birth of Olivia

My name is Sara and I'm 31 years old, my husband Greg and I decided to try and get pregnant as soon as we bought our new home. I've always wanted to be a mother, but the thought of labour terrified me. Coming from Brazil where caesareans are more common than natural birth, even before being pregnant, I had in mind that I would only be able to do it if it was a caesarean. Then after hearing about the benefits of a vaginal labour, I started to consider it, I was still terrified, but willing to try. At some point during my pregnancy I was sure I would die from the pain, silly I know, but that was how scared I was. For the first 5 months I refused to watch any labour video, or research about anything related to that. As I wouldn't have my Mum around, I hired a Brazilian doula to support me during this time and make me feel more secure when giving birth. It was the best decision I ever made, she introduced me to hypnobirthing and only then I started to be more interested in learning what would happen during labour. The first birth video I watched was totally different than the screaming scenes from movies and TV shows I'd seen before, I was so relieved that giving birth could be a pleasant experience. So I started to prepare for it, I learnt everything I could to apply hypnobirthing techniques, I listened to words of affirmation every night with my husband, I visualised my birth and in my mind it would be as positive as it could be. There was one word of affirmation that was always stuck in my mind: *"I can calmly face whatever turn my birthing takes."* My birth preference was to be as natural as possible and if I could cope

14

with the surges I wouldn't get any pain relief. I went from being scared of dying to excited to give birth.

It was the weekend, one week prior to my due date, as we were renovating the house, I was rushing Greg to get our bedroom ready, we still had to put our bed together and buy a couple of things from IKEA. On Saturday afternoon I had a bloody show, I contacted my doula just to let her know, but in my mind I would still have a few days before the labour started. We went shopping and tried to finish a few things in the house. In the early hours of Sunday, Olivia, my baby girl, wasn't moving, so we went to the hospital. Everything was just fine, I had a few contractions, but nothing that I felt concerned about. I had a midwife appointment on Monday morning, she examined me and again, everything was fine. I came back home and went to sleep for a little while. I started to feel some contractions in my back but didn't think much of it, until I went to the bathroom and the rest of my bloody show came. From there the surges started to intensify and I knew Olivia would be born that day. Around midday, I asked my husband to tell his boss it was happening and started to prepare the house, putting some music on, turning on the lavender filled humidifier, I let my doula know so she could come over. By the time she arrived, my contractions were pretty regular. I really wanted to have a natural birth and as much as I knew pain was relative, I wasn't expecting the intensity of mine, so I used the TENS machine at home for as long as I could. Greg and I were sure we would stay at home for quite some time, but thanks to our doula we went to the hospital just in time. The atmosphere of the birth center was amazing, the midwives supporting me were incredible and I felt really calm and secure. My waters broke around 5.30pm just an hour after arriving at the hospital, Olivia had poo'd inside me and the midwives started to assess if I may need to go to the labour ward, I could see they were making an effort to follow my birth preferences and if ever I felt scared about any of the procedures, I asked all the BRAIN questions and they were more than happy to answer. I was 5cm dilated and bleeding more than normal so an obstetrician was called and she identified my placenta was separating from my womb too quickly. With the meconium, excessive bleeding, Olivia being distressed and dilatation not progressing, my alternative was to go for a caesarean. They explained why they recommended it, I once again asked all the questions I needed to make an informed decision, and I agreed to go for the surgery and told the obstetrician that I was using hypnobirthing techniques, she told me to bring any music I would like to the room, unfortunately I was so caught up with everything that I forgot about it! The midwives who were with me from the beginning, also went up to the labour ward, one of them, called Sarah, held me tight in her arms, cuddling me while I was getting the anesthetic, it was the most comforting gesture I could have at that moment, although I was in a surgery room, full of doctors and bright lights I still felt secure.

Olivia was born on Monday 8th November 2021 at 7.05pm. The procedure was very quick and after they checked her, she was put right back on my chest for as long as I wished. Having a caesarean wasn't my first choice but because of hypnobirthing I was able to calmly face the changes my birth took, it was the most amazing experience I have ever had, she is beautiful and the love of my life. If anything, I hope she can have a positive experience as much as I did, if she decides to become a mother.

Sara and baby Olivia

The birth of Darcey

My husband and I attended our hypnobirthing course at around 25 weeks pregnant. Being a yoga teacher I went in open minded and ready to train my mind and body to have the most natural birth we possibly could. My husband is a "scientific fact" person, so he walked into the room a little less open to the idea of "hypno" birthing. That changed within a matter of a morning, and three beautiful (and very different) births later he (and myself) are huge advocates for hypnobirthing.

There was so much we didn't know about birth, we were about to enter into the single most important day(s) that either of us will ever have in our lives, and we wanted to be as prepared and "in the know" as possible.

Darcey's birth, started at home at 41+5, we had a birth pool set up in the lounge of our tiny London flat, and the community midwives were called out a few time's to observe. After 24 hours of being in the first stages of labour, we transferred in to hospital for some help, which was due to the fact I had sickness, which could have quickly led to dehydration. I tried really hard to not be disheartened by transferring into hospital, and when we arrived my waters were broken for me which were meconium stained, meaning I would have had to have transferred in regardless of my own sickness. Mentally I had prepared myself for the idea of this happening, and once I settled with my music, and breathing, we created the perfect hypnobirthing space. I continued to labour for another 12 hours but Darcey's head was not in the optimal position, mixed with both of our heart rates being a little on the high side and the length of labour it was decided a trial of forceps which led to a caesarean was the best route for the both of us. Even though this was not the plan or birth we had wanted, each stage of labour we felt that we had the appropriate knowledge to make a calm, well thought out decision on the next step. I look back on Darcey's birth as incredibly wonderful and hypnobirthing really helped me experience it this way.

Marie and baby Darcey

HOME BIRTH

The birth of Amelie

My second daughter was due just 21 months after my first. My first birth had started at home (with the intention of staying there) but had eventually moved to the hospital for an assisted delivery. Although still a positive experience, this time I was determined to give birth at home.

A week before my due date, my husband, me and our daughter had been at a child's birthday party. I had felt enormous and joked about jumping on the bouncy castle to try and get labour started. We got home around 4pm and at 5pm I was sitting on the sofa and I felt some water trickle down my leg. I had just been for a wee so didn't think it could be this, could it be my waters? I went to the toilet and the water kept coming. I informed my husband who suggested I rest and I went upstairs to lie on my bed for a while.

After about an hour, my surges had not started and my midwife informed me I should head to the hospital to double check it is my waters. Reluctantly I went, I was there for a few hours and they did confirm it was my waters.

We headed back home to wait for my surges to start, grabbing some food and supplies on the way back.

I went straight to bed and not long after my surges started. I tried to sleep but couldn't so just lied on my side doing my breathing. About 2am I woke my husband as I needed to move so we headed downstairs, I put Friends on the TV and sat on my birthing ball doing my breathing.

After another couple of hours my surges had really picked up and I needed a midwife to come out to me. My husband rang them and they soon arrived. Before they offered me any gas and air they sat and watched me to assess how far they thought I was. After around 10 minutes they declared that I was likely in active labour (haha!) and offered me some gas and air which I took. My husband started to fill up the birth pool while I tried to remain conformable.

I found that I couldn't get comfortable anywhere apart from on my back, so lied on the sofa and the midwife offered me a vaginal exam. I accepted and I was fully dilated and told to listen to my body and push if I needed to. My husband quit filling the pool and raced to my side. After 2 very short pushes (my body doing the pushing), my daughter Amelie was born onto the sofa.

I was so happy I got my home birth and although I didn't get to use the pool, it was completely perfect. I often wish I could go back and do it again and I have hypnobirthing to thank for that!

Claire and baby Amelie

The birth of Theo

I was "due" on October 19th 2021, but on Thursday September 30th 2021, I went into early labor.

We knew it was possible that he would come early because of a number of things, but he actually ended up arriving RIGHT at 38 weeks!

So Thursday afternoon, September 30th I had what's called a "bloody show," and then immediately began early labor contractions. Honestly,g they just felt like period cramps, so I figured it could be a few weeks yet and maybe false labor. Little did I know!

The contractions never stopped, and Friday at work, I lost my mucus plug throughout the day. The contractions were a bit more intense but still what I would call moderate period cramps.

Again, I was in denial and thought I still had a good 2 weeks left. We happened to have a prenatal appointment that afternoon and the midwives agreed that it was too early to know if it would end up being true labor or not.

I didn't sleep well, and on Saturday morning our sweet doula stopped by and we talked for a bit. We both agreed that it was PROBABLY close to baby time, but still could last a few days.

At this point my contractions were uncomfortable to the point of having to breathe through some of them and stop walking occasionally. I could fake it pretty well in front of other people though, and...well...Saturday afternoon I got it in my head that I MUST meal prep frozen meals. So hubby and I went to Whole Foods and then meal prepped almost

10 full meals while I was in early labor. Again, I woke up with every contraction that night, and they were anywhere from 5-10 minutes apart consistently.

Sunday came around and I was definitely uncomfortable at this point. I had to stop and lean over the couch or counter with each contraction, we were home all day trying to relax, going through the Miles Circuit, and taking occasional warm baths.

Oh, and an interesting tidbit—my contractions were almost always five minutes apart. From Thursday, all the way until Theo was born. Sometimes they would go back to 15 minutes apart or so, but mostly they stayed around 5 minutes apart. And even in full-on labor they were never closer than 4-5 minutes! So weird!

So Sunday night around 7pm we called our doula and midwife. At this point I was working hard to practice my hypnobirthing breathing, keeping my body relaxed during contractions, and vocalising through the particularly uncomfortable ones. Out of all the techniques I learned in hypnobirthing, the breathing and relaxed jaw was the most helpful for me and something I used all the way through.

Our birth team arrived around 7.45pm. I told my midwife I wanted to be checked, but I didn't want to know how far along I was because I was afraid that if I was barely dilated it would make me feel super defeated and tired. So she planned to check me and just give me suggestions to continue labor. BUT, then she checked me and said "if it's an exciting number do you want to know?" I was like "yes!" I was dilated to a 6cm! I was officially in active labor!

THANK GOD. After laboring since Thursday, I cried when she told me that. I was so relieved!

For the next 12 hours I went for a walk with Russ and our doula, we walked up and down the stairs, I spent time laboring in the tub and on the toilet (which is surprisingly one of the best places to breathe baby down!) and I tried to sleep in between contractions.

Another interesting piece was that I never had a big "transition" period. Sometime early morning I began to feel nauseated during contractions and was feeling super fatigued, probably around 6.30-7am or so.

We tried breathing, peppermint oil, lying in bed, etc. and my body was beginning to push by itself during contractions. They were very intense and I had been vocalising through them most of the night. So I think that time period was my "transition," even though my contractions still stayed around 5-7 minutes apart.

At 8am or so I told our midwives that I was starting to lose steam and was struggling. I was exhausted from barely sleeping, the contractions were super intense, and I had been in labor a LONG time.

Our midwife checked me one more time and said that his head was literally RIGHT inside. So I had breathed him down all the way and he was just hanging out. She had me go back to the toilet to labor a bit more and push with my body to bring him down to crowning.

I spent just a few minutes there, my body was pushing on its own, so I pushed with it, and honestly I thought man he's GOT to be crowning now. Not quite, it took a few good contractions before he was actually there.

They had me go to the tub at this point because I wanted to bring Theo into the world in the water!

The intensity was kind of surprising to me, to be honest. There was SO much pressure and there were definitely a couple of moments that I thought wow, how is this doable?! But my doula and midwives were so good about telling me to keep from tensing up and clenching my jaw.

Russ was there right beside me, ready to catch Theo when he appeared, and it took just 12 minutes of pushing for him to appear! His head took a few contractions to come out, and everyone started exclaiming about how much hair he had! I wasn't able to speak but I thought, "wait, I didn't have heartburn! How does he have hair?!"

Russ said as his head came out, Theo was facing down, and the coolest thing is that babies turn as they enter the world. So as soon as his head came out, within the same contraction I pushed the rest of his body out (way easier than his head!) and Russ could see him turn mid-way through so he came out the rest of the way face-up!

Russ caught baby Theo as he came out and Russ lifted him out of the water. One of the coolest moments for us both! He brought Theo to me and put him in my arms and he started crying.

I felt such shock and surprise at how fast that part of the birth was. After days of laboring, it was just incredible! I actually said "oh my gosh, it's a baby!!"

He had so much vernix on him, and he was perfectly pink and wrinkly and adorable. It was the absolute wildest feeling to finally see the sweet baby that had been growing inside me for so long. It's a feeling I just cannot put into words.

We moved to the bed to birth the placenta, and it was kind of a whirlwind of things after that. Theo latched and began nursing immediately and he did so good, I was so proud of him!!

We weighed him, took his measurements, and all in our bedroom! Then our sweet midwives made an herbal bath for me and Theo, and I was able to spend time in a bath with him, nursing again.

It was the most incredible, wild, intense thing I have ever experienced. I am so thankful that we were able to do a home water birth, and Russ and I still talk about it today and how amazing it was to do it together.

So thankful for our doula, our midwives, and for our sweet Theo. He truly is a gift from God, as his name means.

Lexi and baby Theo

The birth of Phoebe

The night that Phoebe was born and the way in which it happened will stay with me for the rest of my life in a way no other experience so far in my life will.

During my pregnancy, I had been lucky to find out about hypnobirthing and had started doing the occasional meditation and deep breathing exercise from about 25 weeks onwards. I read some great hypnobirthing books and really looked forward to the new 'The Hypnobirthing Podcast' episodes of positive birth stories that would come out every few weeks. When I first got pregnant, I genuinely thought that the only decision I needed to make about birth was 'epidural or no epidural' and I had no idea what happened in my body during birth. Hypnobirthing and how it brings us back to our heritage of natural birth without fear blew my mind- how had I made it to 27 years old without knowing all this history and never being told how my uterus worked??

After the initial amazement, it didn't take long for me to decide on a homebirth. I kept an open mind however, as all the stats seemed to suggest that most first time mums transfer into hospital during a homebirth. As the due date drew close I had a few doubts- could I do it? How high was my pain threshold? Had I practiced my breathing enough? But I also thought, however she arrived, I would be at peace with it.

On December 9th, I had mild contractions all day, which built in intensity and were about 5 minutes apart when I went to bed. But overnight they calmed down and things were back to normal in the morning. However, from 10am on December 10th they started again and I was pretty sure they weren't going anywhere. I walked the dog, tidied up a bit and my husband called my Mum that she should come over around 4pm that day. I had been told not to call the midwives until the contractions were 3 minutes apart. This seemed to take forever, but did speed up quite a bit after my waters broke around 5.30pm. I was so lucky to have both my Mum and husband by my side. I laboured in the living room by the fireplace, over my birth ball and rocked from side to side as it felt so nice on my back. My Mum held my hands through the contractions and Peter pressed on my back. I used a TENS machine and paracetamol for pain relief, and that was doing a pretty good job! What surprised me was how helpful it was that my Mum kept reminding me to breathe- I focused on my breath with each contraction and before I knew it, it was over.

Although before going into labour I had prepared candles, fairy lights and affirmation cards, in the end, I was in another zone and hardly noticed any of my surroundings really. I said affirmations in my head: 'no surge is stronger than me because it is me', 'my surges are strong because I am strong' and 'I am a birthing warrior'. The midwives were called around 9pm, but took over an hour to get to us, by which point I had moved to our bedroom and had kindly been undressed by my Mum and Peter (not very glamourous, but I left my fuzzy socks and jumper on!).

I will not go into detail of the midwives involvement. Although they were lovely, they brought a whole level of medicalisation and fear into a process which was going very smoothly. Fortunately, I was in the zone and even when they called the paramedics (why they thought it was practical to transfer me after one slightly lower baby heartbeat while I was 10cm dilated remains beyond me- no doubt I would have given birth in the ambulance) it didn't throw me off. After moving onto all fours and a few strong pushes, Phoebe was born at 00:50 am on December 11th, on our bed (the same place she was made, what a wonderful circle of life) and I was so proud. Looking around the room, at my Mum and Peter, I was so happy she was there safe and that I did it at home. That ecstatic feeling has stayed with me ever since the birth. The cord was clamped, Peter cut it and then I put her on my chest and she fed! What an amazing feeling, to see the face of the tiny human being you have been growing for 9 months on the inside, now outside and having their first meal!

I feel it is so important to share this story with others, because although I did the prep work, researched the process of birth and had 'a plan', the medical professionals I encountered saw homebirth as a nice option, but were never that encouraging. The chances of a first time mum (albeit low risk) doing this seemed slim as well, given the evidence I had seen about transfer rates. But I truly feel that if I can do it, anyone can. I had no pain relief other than the TENS machine and paracetamol- I had gas and air after the birth as I needed a few stitches and that is powerful stuff! The whole experience has taught me I can do what I put my mind to, and that has given me so much energy in the first month postpartum, despite a lack of sleep and constantly breastfeeding.

I believe if more women had this kind of birth experience, surrounded by loving birth partners and believed in their innate ability to birth, the start of motherhood would be much smoother and gentler for them as well. I feel so passionately about this that I am about to start training as a hypnobirthing instructor- with the goal of becoming a doula that supports women throughout their journey to motherhood.

Lizzie and baby Phoebe

The birth of Daniel

Coming from Greece, I always used to hear stories about women giving birth through scheduled caesarean for no valid reason (I have even heard of stories of women whose doctors scheduled them in before their due date because the doctors would go on vacation). Also, giving birth at home is extremely rare and I grew up to believe that "you must be crazy" to give birth at home. Or "poor her she didn't make it in time to the hospital, she gave birth at home". So naturally I was not comfortable with this idea either.

However, in The Netherlands, where we currently live, home births are very common. I believed that my pregnancy and how I would give birth was a choice to be made by the doctor following my pregnancy, as in Greece, antenatal care is primarily OBG-led, and there are midwives who act sort of like nurses during labour.

However, in The Netherlands the antenatal care is midwife-led, and you only get to see an OBG in case there is medical concern during the pregnancy; then your midwife will refer you to the OBG.

This and the fact that 30% of Dutch women give birth at home scared me in the beginning.

During our first appointment with the midwives, I remember I told them almost in panic "I want a physiological birth, not caesarean and definitely not at home". Little did I know that home birth would become scenario A in my birth preferences.

I think that the way our midwives approached us in each appointment played a very big role in how my mindset started to shift. During each appointment, they would just ask me how I am feeling, how my days are going and if I have any complaints. They were really relaxed, and they didn't treat me like I was sick. They would always answer all my questions, even the most stupid ones and ease my worries.

The pregnancy was progressing smoothly, I was feeling great, so early on I decided that if everything kept going smoothly, I wouldn't take any time off from my maternity leave before my due date.

While I was reading my antenatal books (*"The Mama Natural Week-By-Week Guide to Pregnancy and Childbirth"* by Genevieve Howland & *"How to Grow a Baby and Push It Out: Your No-nonsense Guide to Pregnancy and Birth"* by Clemmie Hooper) I started learning more about the physiology of birth and that was the first time that I came across the term "hypnobirthing". That's when the seed for a home birth was also planted.

One day, I came across a video of a labouring woman in Greece, giving birth in a labour ward. The way the attending doctor (quite famous) was talking to the woman sounded really off to me (sort of diminishing); then, when the baby was born, the nurse showed the baby to the woman and while she reached to take the baby in her arms, the nurses took the baby away for a wash before returning to mom (needless to say that the baby was crying desperately all this time). This whole visual broke my heart; I didn't know what hit me and I started crying like a baby; maybe the hormones, maybe I got emotional from the whole birth; one thing I knew for sure: I wouldn't want that for me.

And then I discovered The Hypnobirthing Podcast and Instagram page which shared a video of a home birth which hit right home! I started crying again but this time filled with happiness, and I remembered I showed the video to my husband, Hugo, and I told him "that's what I want for us".

In the beginning he was skeptical but after a few talks he was fully on board, which was very important to me... to feel that he was in this with me, that he supported my decision, that he also wanted the same.

So, we started the preparations for our homebirth early on, I think when I was around 24 weeks. Hypnobirthing course, breathing exercises, massage techniques, ordering a birthing pool etc.

We also arranged for a birth photographer, Inge Berken, which even though I was a bit skeptical about in the beginning (would one more stranger in the room be conducive to my environment?), it was one of the best decisions we made and of course money well spent. You see, I wanted to capture these moments so that we can look back to them, but I also wanted both Hugo and I to be focused on what would be going on with me and the baby and not having to think about taking pictures.

Plus, since we live alone in NL and our families are far away, we thought it would be the best way to make them feel "present" at the birth of their grandchild & nephew. I know that everyone would like to be there with us, but most of all, my mother.

On Sunday, August 15th, it was a nice summer day, so Hugo and I spent the whole day at the beach.

While we were there enjoying the warm sun, I was reading the news and the weather forecast for the upcoming week and I read that upcoming Saturday, August 21st, would be the last summery warm and sunny day of the year, and since the Dutch summer is nothing but a disgrace to the word "summer", I decided that I wanted to grasp every opportunity I have to enjoy the sun before the baby comes.

So, I went ahead and booked a nice breakfast for us by the beach to have our coffee and enjoy the day under the sun.

Around this time, Hugo had a call with his mother to check on how we were doing. During this call, Hugo turned to me, and asked if I know when the next full moon would be, and I replied to him that it would be on August 22nd but why would he be asking; he didn't give me a reason and he returned to the call with his mother.

You see, his mother is quite an intuitive woman and once they hung up, I asked him if his mother said anything about the baby being born with a full moon and replied "no, she just said we need to be alert and read the signs".

Almost every night during these days, I would go over several details with Hugo, to make sure we are on the same boat: which essential oils and what music I would like, what he needs to do, what he needs to offer and not ask (e.g. if I didn't eat, he would just bring me something instead of asking if I want to eat), his massage techniques and pressure points and our safe word.

I know how worried he can get, so one night we sat down and I told him: "there might come a time during labor that I might say that I can't do it anymore or that I don't want to do it anymore. You will not give in. If I indeed feel like I want to go to the hospital, I will look in the eye and say: now it is time to go to the hospital. Anything even slightly different than this doesn't count".

And we would go over our plan again: he would come into the pool with me, he would be the one to greet the baby and hold him.

It's now Saturday, August 21st and I am 39 weeks. I woke up quite early at around 8am because we had to be by the beach at 10am for our breakfast reservation and we wanted to avoid all the traffic. I was really excited for the day but, to my surprise, it wasn't that sunny as forecasted; on the contrary it was gloomy and cloudy and even foggy, but I wouldn't let anything ruin my mood and I was determined that we go to the beach no matter what.

I went to the bathroom to get ready and that's when I noticed some period like staining, I called the midwives because I wasn't sure what was going on. As it turns out I had lost my mucus plug, the midwife told me it was normal, nothing to worry about, I should go on with my day as planned and if anything changes, I should give them a call again. So off we went to the beach, had our nice breakfast as the weather started turning lovely; sunny, not as warm as we thought it would get but still pleasant to be by the beach.

We stayed there till early in the afternoon or so, and in the ride back home, I started feeling quite tired, like after a long trip, a bit drowsy and like something had upset my stomach.

We arrived home but we still had some grocery shopping to do, so I told Hugo I would like to walk to the grocery store, as I wasn't feeling like going back in the car and I preferred to walk so that some fresh air would hit my face and he would come meet me there with the car to bring the groceries back home. At the grocery store while I shopped, I started thinking of what I would like to eat during labor, so I bought a bunch of mini carrots, ice lollies and cereal bars. (With hindsight, mini carrots are a terrible idea to chew on mid surge.)

It was around 5.30pm, just right after having put all the groceries away when I started feeling some cramps. Nothing intense, just some noticeable pinches. I told Hugo and he seemed really calm about it. We were planning to do a "before- after" type of picture by drawing a bomb on my belly for the "before part" so we decided that this was a really good time to do it. Hugo started drawing the bomb on my belly and then he whispered "Bebe, Benifca is playing tonight. Please let papa watch the game" (you see our papa is a big football fan). I looked at him and smiled and said, "Oh don't worry, he will". We took the pictures and off I went to the shower to get the crayon off my belly.

While I was in the shower, I kept thinking "Is this it??? Or maybe not?? Nah... maybe not". Even though the shower was refreshing, I was still feeling a bit under the weather, and I decided to lie down to take a nap. I woke up after an hour or so as I felt the cramps getting more intense.

I walked downstairs and lied on the couch while Hugo was preparing dinner. We had a lovely dinner of steaks while watching the football match. Thankfully Benfica won, so our papa was in a really good mood.

During the game at around 8.30pm, my cramps turned into surges coming and going so I decided to give a call again to my midwives and let them know what was going on.

I was glad to hear that Caresse picked up, the one of our midwives' who I felt the most comfortable with. She asked me how long each surge lasted and how far apart they were, but I couldn't tell as I was not monitoring them. I had read that constantly monitoring with an app how far apart the surges are will not do you any good, it is more likely to have an opposite effect.

But I couldn't focus on counting how many breaths I was taking or ask Hugo to monitor every time a surge was coming.

So I gave in and downloaded an app and at 9.30pm I started monitoring. I was sitting on my birthing ball as it was feeling more comfortable than the couch and after the game finished, we put the US version of The Office on, as it is maybe my favorite series of all times.

At this point, the surges lasted 30-60 seconds, approximately 10 minutes apart and I could still talk through them. Occasionally, I would get an intense one that would last 90-120 seconds but the next one wouldn't come for 15-20 minutes. At around 11pm we decided to go lie down in bed to get some rest. Hugo seemed a bit more worried at this point as my surges were getting more intense, but I convinced him to get some sleep since they were not consistent and when I felt the need, I would wake him up.

While Hugo was drifting away, during every surge I would focus on my breathing and after it was gone, I would be returning to texting my mother giving her a full "report", as I knew that she was terribly anxious being 2860km away and that was the only way to keep her anxiety under control and make the distance feel shorter.

In the meantime, I was also in contact with our birth photographer, Inge, in order to keep her in the loop and for her to be ready to come over when needed.

For the next 2 hours the surges would get much more intense but still not consistent. Every time a surge was coming, I would wake up to hit the app and monitor. During every surge I would stand up and bend over with the elbows against the bed, moving my hips left and right until the surge has passed. During some surges though, the very intense ones, I was feeling the need to go and sit on the toilet, and I ended up spending quite some time in the bathroom, as every time I would get up from the toilet, another surge would come.

At this point, the trick with the comb came in handy. I have to say that this tricks is a miracle and from the moment I grabbed the combs (one in each hand) I wouldn't take a step without them.

So, it was around 1am and apart from a few catnaps, I hadn't got any sleep as I was too occupied monitoring with the app and so I told myself "enough is enough you need to sleep, if the baby is coming you will know". I took a shower, I informed my Mom and Inge that I will try to get some sleep so that they don't get worried, I put my phone on 'do not disturb', laid in bed and magically got 2.5 hours of sleep in.

The rest of the night went on like this, catnapping followed by a myriad of trips to the bathroom and bending over the bed to breathe through the surges.

At around 6.30am, I decided to take another shower and head downstairs to the living room since it was clear that I wouldn't be sleeping any longer. I woke Hugo up and we both headed downstairs and lied on the couch as the sun was coming up.

I managed to sleep a bit further till 8.30am or so, when I woke up to an intense surge, and decided to give a call to our midwifes to give them an update. Our midwife, Caresse, asked me if she should come over already so that we could do a check. I explained to her how the surges were still inconsistent but very intense and we both decided that I would give her a call again when I felt that she should come over. We spent the next couple of hours with me sitting on the birthing ball and Hugo tending to my every need (bringing me snacks, water, massaging) and preparing the space.

As the surges were still inconsistent, I decided to call the midwife again at around 11am and ask her to come over because I needed to know where I was standing. After 10 minutes or so, the doorbell rang and Caresse was there. She felt my belly, checked the heartbeat of the baby and how far dilated I was; 4cm. Then she told me that everything looks really good, but since the contractions were not consistent, she would like to come back in 2 hours and check me gain. She then advised me that if in 2 hours, there was no change to how my contractions were going, she'd like to break my waters, as this could cause a change to the contractions. Even though I was really tired, I really wanted to avoid going to the hospital, so I asked her to tell me what would happen if after breaking the waters there wouldn't be any change, as I needed to discuss with Hugo and take a decision in case we need to turn to plan B.

She explained, and we agreed that she will come back in 2 hours. To be honest, I don't remember much of what happened in those 2 hours. I remember that we put up the pool in our living room and that I almost choked on a baby carrot, because a contraction came while my mouth was full and I had to spit everything out in order to breath

Two hours went by and at 1pm Caresse came back. We all went upstairs so that she could examine me and since nothing had really changed we decided to break the membranes. Breaking the membranes was a very weird and funny sensation; I felt a pinch and then I started "leaking" uncontrollably; I laid waiting for the flow to stop, but when I stood up a big gush of water came out.

While I was lying in the bed, Caresse asked Hugo to start filling the pool and let our birth photographer know that she should be on her way. So, Hugo went downstairs to continue with his "tasks" and I stayed in bed a little longer. Then I decided to take another shower to relax, and I hopped in while Caresse headed downstairs to assist Hugo, call the attending nurse and prepare the scene.

I don't know for how long I was in that shower, but when I went downstairs (felt like a lifetime of going down the stairs; every other step I had to stop and breathe through surges). I saw that everybody had come in and had already taken their places; Dam, the nurse, was assisting Caresse; Inge, our photographer, was arranging her lenses; and Hugo was setting up the last details (my clary sage and lavender, the twinkly lights, music on, water and snack next to the pool and my combs in grabbing distance) waiting for me.

I was really looking forward to hopping into that pool, as at this point, my contractions were very intense, and I could only find relief in the water along with Hugo's light touch massage. As I submerged myself into the pool, I fell deep into my bubble.

Breathing and repeating mantras in my head:
Floppy face floppy fanny
My baby, my partner and I are a team
We are meeting our baby today

With every surge we are breathe, we are closer to welcoming our baby

The surges are not stronger than me because they are me

Knees in Calves Out.

With every surge, everything around me would get muffled, the room would become silent and distant. The only person I could feel and hear was Hugo. He was there next to me, calm, with his gentle touch, whispering and encouraging me.

And after every surge I would come back, Caresse would ask me very gently to stand a bit out of the water so that she can check the heartbeat of the baby. She could do it fast & I would return into my bubble. After some time, she also asked me to come out of the pool so that she could check how far I was.

When I went back in the pool (this time with Hugo joining me in the pool), Caresse told me that I might feel a need to push but I shouldn't push just yet. After a few minutes, I felt that need but I also felt that Caresse was not in the room (which she wasn't) so I remember yelling "Caresse I have to push!!!" and I heard her from the hallway saying "Ok!"

From that point on, I remember everything like haze, being very fast and very slow at the same time; yet very vivid. With every surge, I was trying to guide by breath down and the baby out. After every breath, the pressure was getting higher, so the breathing turned into roaring.

After several pushes, I could feel the head of the baby coming almost out and then back in, I felt like my breath was not long enough and I told Hugo "I can't do this!", and he, as calm as ever, said "You got this! You are doing it!"

So I gave the next pushes my everything and pushed myself like I've never pushed myself before.

Now after every push, I am asking "Is he out? Is he out?" and Hugo and Caresse almost in unison said "almost! Let's do one more push"

And then, one final long roar, Caresse saying "come on, come on, come on" and Hugo saying "Opah... opah... opah..." in a tearful voice and our little boy was earthbound, he gently glided into the water onto his papas arms.

5.35pm, and his name: Daniel Odysseas. Our little baby Ody.

Hugo with tears in his eyes caught him and brought him very slowly and gently out of the water, onto his chest, while I was trying to catch my breath and turn around.

And there he was, our little boy, so small, so fragile, so lovely, so perfect. And there we were, finally the three of us, all together in the pool.

I was feeling so overwhelmingly powerful, proud, happy, emotional and ecstatic.

I forgot immediately about any pain that I felt the last 24 hours and we stayed there in the pool the three of us and time stood still. I couldn't get enough of him. His little hands, his little feet, and his big black eyes, so awake and so aware of everything around him. We stayed in the pool until the cord stopped pulsating and then Hugo cut it while baby was laying quietly on my chest.

Then after that, Caresse told me that we have been quite some time in the pool and that she would like to pull the placenta, as me being in the water, she couldn't estimate if I was bleeding and how much, and it would be best that I go on dry land. I agreed with her, gave one push for the placenta to be born, and I went out of the pool as I was starting to feel quite cold as well.

Baby and Papa stayed in the pool to enjoy some skin to skin while mama went to lay on the couch. I was trembling like a fish and I couldn't tell if it was because I was cold or the adrenaline, seems it was a bit of both.

I lied there while Caresse gave me 2 stitches and after she was finished, I got the baby back in my arms, for some skin to skin and to start trying to get a latch. He was so tiny he could barely grab my boob, but after a few tries, we managed to establish our first latch and he ate a bit.

And while we lied there, the video calls started flowing in. First my family, my parents, and my siblings and then Hugo's family, his parents, his sister and his firstborn. I will never forget the feeling; a storm of emotions; happiness and pride showing our families who we have created, excitement and happy tears from their side seeing their grandson for the first time; and a small cloud of light sadness over all of us, as I believe that we all wanted to be all together for this first meeting and not over a video, and we all knew that it will be some time until they get to meet him in person.

After some time passed, we ate the Dutch customary treat "beschuit met muisjes" (a biscuit with a thick layer of butter and sprinkled blue and white sugarcoated anise seeds) and the time for the first checks arrived. Caresse performed all necessary actions, weighing, measuring, reflex checking and vitamin K.

And then we dressed him, the clothes we chose for him as his first outfit was the same outfit that Hugo wore as his first, as his mom was kind enough to give this to us (I see a little tradition being born here.)

It must have already been around 8pm when everybody left, and we were finally the 3 of us. We cuddled on the couch, eating pizza, savoring every minute, every sound and move that the baby was making; he was so small so fragile, yet both Hugo and I felt like we knew him since forever.

Before I close this story, I would like to give a shout out to all the birth partners out there, as they are the safeguards of the birthing environment, but an extra super-duper gigantic one to MY amazing birth partner, Hugo. Without him, I don't believe I would have had the blessing of going through this experience. He was there, so invested in his role and tasks, next to me, to us.

It was important to me that he would be not only present but an active participant to the birth of our son; and God knows how important it was for him that I wanted him there involved too; I like to think that the birth of Ody was, in a way, healing.

Nefeli and baby Daniel Odysseas

The birth of Abel

When I fell pregnant with my second child I found myself feeling overwhelmed when I thought about having to give birth again. I hadn't realised that my first birth experience had left me with doubt in my ability to do it "successfully". I spoke with my sister who had her first child a few months earlier and she told me that she had done hypnobirthing and leant me a book. I read the book, did a hypnobirthing course, a yoga course and listened to The Hypnobirthing Podcast that was recommended by another friend. Well, I went into this birth with all the knowledge I could find and it really helped. Knowledge is powerful. I felt so sure in what I had learnt this time we decided to opt for a homebirth knowing that if I changed my mind on the day I could go into hospital.

The day before my due date at 12.30am I felt movement in my body, I knew it could take some time from my previous pregnancy and as my contractions weren't that strong I tried to get some rest. At 2am they were a lot stronger, so I decided to do some wiggling over the birth ball and came downstairs as we had more space. At 3.30am we rang for the midwife as I was so relaxed in my own home that I didn't want to leave. At 4am I knew there was a change in me as my waters broke and from everything I had done before, it helped me understand that change. At 4.30am the midwife arrived, I remember shouting that I was doing a poo and the midwife basically threw all her equipment into the house and rang for the second midwife and within minutes I started breathing my baby out. I did decide at the very last minute I wanted to be laying so hopped onto the sofa and at 4.45am, my beautiful baby boy was here.

By 7am the midwives had left and we were at home all settled on the sofa with tea, toast and the TV, nursing a very hungry boy. It was the most amazing experience to be at home and so calming. I really believe that without doing the hypnobirthing and all the other bits of learning I would not have been so calm and would have never been motivated to even book in a home birth. It was a truly magical experience.

Tayla and baby Abel

HOSPITAL BIRTH

The birth of Elle

When I was first pregnant with my daughter I often imagined how my birth would be, and probably like many others, my head was filled with images of me on my back, on a hospital bed, screaming and feeling out of control. This sounded horrible and I knew I wanted different. This is when I discovered hypnobirthing. My husband and I attended a hypnobirthing class when I was at the end of my second trimester and loved it. The theories and teachings were so logical and made us feel so excited about our upcoming birth. Before the course I was adamant I would never want a home birth, but after learning about the body and the mind and how birth works, I changed my mind and started planning for my home birth.

My daughter was due just after Christmas and on Boxing Day I woke at 4am with some light bleeding. I wasn't sure what this meant so thought the safest thing to do would be to head to the hospital to be checked. Whilst there, they informed me my cervix was nicely closed still (not something I really wanted to hear) and that the bleeding could have been down to thrush (although I never had any symptoms of this so to this day I am still not sure if this is what it was). While we were still in the hospital, I started to feel some light surges but because I wanted to give birth at home, I didn't mention it out of fear of not being able to leave.

We were discharged and once back home by surges ramped up. I was using my breathing techniques and a birth ball to help.

Around 7.30am a midwife came out to us and asked if she could do a vaginal exam, I consented and she informed me I was around 4cms and in active labour, so she would be staying. My husband filled the birthing pool and I got in – it was utter bliss.

My labour was long, I was in the pool for hours and hours and saw around 4 different midwives because of shift changes. For the many hours I was in labour, I was just used my breathing, the birth pool and gas and air to help me through.

After a while I got out of the pool and stayed on dry land. Around 12am the next day, they told me I was fully dilated. The second stage of my labour lasted 2 hours, baby's head kept appearing and then disappearing (which is normal, but not much progress was being made). I was exhausted, I had been awake for 30 hours at this point, baby was exhausted and starting to show signs for stress and so the decision was made to transfer to the hospital for some assistance. I used my BRAIN tool to assess my options and work out what was best for me and baby and I was happy with this decision. We went by ambulance which was fine and as soon as we arrived at the hospital I was taken to a delivery room and offered an episiotomy and forceps. Again, using my BRAIN tool I agreed to both and within about 10 minutes my daughter was born.

I always say, on paper my birth probably looks horrible. Long labour, ambulance ride and an episiotomy and forceps. But I can't stress enough how positive I feel about it. Because of hypnobirthing and the skills I gained, I was able to stay in control of my decisions and only agree to things I felt happy with. I look back at my first labour with such wonderful memories and I feel like a total badass for managing my way through such a long labour.

Claire and baby Elle

The birth of Felix

When our antenatal class got cancelled, we were looking for another way to prepare ourselves for our son's arrival. Having been listening to The Hypnobirthing Podcast, I was absolutely delighted to hear Claire was now offering an Essentials Course as we were only a few weeks away from our due dates.

The course and podcast have been so helpful. They have helped us navigate the UK birthing system, know our options and know how to interpret/challenge what we were told.

My pregnancy was an "easy" one, a little discomfort in the beginning and end. My belly and baby were considered small and we had to have extra ultrasounds to check development. Thanks to the course I was able to distance myself from that and remember I am 5ft, small and my baby would be the right size for my body.

In our birth preferences, we opted for a hospital birth where we would feel both more comfortable and safer. And it was important to me to try a fully natural « dry » birth with the epidural remaining an option if I changed my mind.

I'd been in labour for about a day before heading to hospital and did it all: the bath, the naps, food I enjoyed. I even went to my prenatal yoga class the day before he was born as I wasn't sure whether I was in labour or having braxton hicks!

On the day, we got to the hospital and I was 2cm dilated. I understood what my pain relief options were and opted for morphine to help me manage the pain. Having been in labour for a while, I wanted an epidural to help me manage the discomfort but had to wait to be more dilated. 6 hours after arriving my contractions were getting much stronger and I asked to be checked but the midwives said "that's not how they do it", thankfully my waters broke and they checked me - 5cm. We asked for an anesthetist to have the epidural but they replied they were all in theatre and trying to see if they could get someone. Somehow I knew I wouldn't get the epidural at that point. This is where the hypnobirthing course came in really handy!

I'm a very anxious person but I kept repeating to myself "my surges cannot be stronger than me because they are me" / "every surge brings me closer to meeting my baby" / "I'm a strong and powerful woman, I can do this". By the time we arrived in our labour room about 30 minutes later, I heard the midwife say to a nurse "she's fully dilated so we're going to have to start pushing". And I didn't panic! I got into a zone, tuning in with my body and embracing each sensation to help me understand how we could work together. My midwife was amazing as well, she helped me find a comfortable position, really coached me through it and barely touched me the whole time I was pushing.

I ended up with a beautiful baby boy named Felix who was 51cm and 2.89kg. I had a few natural tears and no need for any instruments or medical support. It made me feel incredibly empowered and absolutely amazed at what my body can do!

I am so thankful for such a positive experience and attribute a lot of it to hypnobirthing. I am absolutely convinced I would not have had the same experience had I not done it.

Clementine and baby Felix

The birth of Eli

Eli is my first baby, and I was blessed with a straight-forward, low-risk pregnancy. I desperately wanted a natural, medication-free birth, but grew up being told I had a low pain threshold, so didn't like my chances. Listening to The Hypnobirthing Podcast was my first introduction to hypnobirthing, and after that I decided to do the course. I loved the versatility of hypnobirthing, and that it focused on educating me, and giving me the skills to be calm, know my options, and play an active role in the birth of my baby, no matter what the circumstances.

My birth preferences highlighted that I had done the hypnobirthing course, but also noted some key things:

I am quite a sensitive person, and value when people are patient with me.

My ideal birth is one where I feel supported, listened-to, and dealt with in an emotionally sensitive way.

Avoid vaginal examinations. If an examination is required, please do not tell me how many cm's I am.

I'm comfortable with traditional terms such as "contractions" and "pushing".

Jared to announce the baby's sex.

Eli was given the 'due date' of Friday 6th February, although being my first birth I was fully prepared to be waiting a further two weeks. On Monday 1st February, I had an appointment with my midwife. She informed me that baby was head down and engaged, and suggested I begin thinking about a stretch and sweep for my next appointment at 40 weeks and 2 days. That afternoon, I started to lose some mucus plug.

On the morning of Wednesday 3rd February, I woke up with some cramping that seemed to come and go in waves. These 'contractions' went on for about 50 seconds, were about 4-5 minutes apart, but were not very painful and disappeared by about midday. In the afternoon I had some more mucus plug and sent my husband a text, "okay, this baby is definitely getting ready to meet us earth side". The same contractions woke me up on Thursday 4th February and had subsided by midday. I did what any first-time mother would do in my situation, and Googled, which suggested that I was likely in early labour. I sent my husband a text saying, "I'm thinking tomorrow will be our day".

And I was right. Soon after going to bed on Thursday night, the contractions started up again. My husband, Jared, was sleeping soundly next to me, but I just couldn't get comfortable. I decided that if this baby really was joining us, it was best for him to get as much rest as possible, so I headed to the living room. I put on my TENS machine and bounced around on my exercise ball for a while. The couch started to look appealing, so I leaned over the backrest on all fours and even managed to nap on and off for a few hours. At around 3am, I went to the toilet only to discover some more mucus plug. I found I needed to go to the toilet pretty frequently after that! At about 4:30am, I woke my husband and reported my frequent toileting, and he suggested I ring the hospital to get their opinion. I spoke to a midwife who said that it was likely I was in early labour and discussed induction on Saturday or Sunday if this continued. The instructions that came with my TENS machine said not to use it while asleep, but I really didn't care at that point, so got into bed and napped! Sometime during my nap, I felt a slight 'pop' and some discharge.

I woke after a few hours and Jared decided it was best he stay home from work today as it didn't seem like these contractions were going to stop. I continued on my exercise ball, crunched some ice and tried to eat some peanut butter toast. I was tracking my contractions on my phone, and by midday they were lasting a minute long, with a 3 minute break, however, every now and then I'd get a 5 minute break, or even an 8 minute break! This totally confused me, and Google had no answers, so we rang the hospital again. They asked a few questions, and suggested we come in for a check, but asked us not to bring bags up, as it was likely we'd be sent home again.

One thing is for certain, contractions in the car are a whole different ball game. It felt impossible to find a good position. We made it up to the maternity ward and a lovely midwife, Sarah, showed us to a room. She took my pad for testing and went in search of a birthing ball for me. When she returned, she confirmed that my waters had broken (probably the 'pop' I felt in the early hours of the morning!), and that I was dehydrated. She also discussed antibiotics given that I was group B strep (GBS) positive, and an induction to get things moving given the risks associated with the GBS infection. This hit me like a brick wall. I was okay with an induction if it was medically necessary, but deep down it felt like a blow given that my body seemed to be on the right track. I told Jared that if I was having an induction, I'd opt for an epidural at the same time. Thankfully Sarah informed is that there were no available beds for inductions at that stage, so I had a little while to process it all.

It felt like Sarah had not long left the room when I started feeling lots of pressure and almost the urge to push.

Sarah returned and introduced me to the midwife, Olivia, who would take over at changeover time. I reported the pressure and urge to push, and Olivia suggested that she do an internal examination. I was happy with this, so got on the bed ready for her to check. I was pretty much in my own world, but in the background heard Olivia say to Jared, "I know her birth preference is to not know how dilated she is, but I think she'll want to hear this", to which Jared obviously gave permission. Olivia gently informed me that I was 9cms dilated and I said, "oh good, I was hoping for 3cms!" Olivia asked Jared to push the nurse call button, as the room was not set up for a delivery yet, and all I remember was a quiet and organised flurry of midwives setting up the room and inserting an IV drip in to address my dehydration. Olivia informed that they would not have a chance to give me antibiotics as baby was well and truly on its way.

Sarah came up to my head, held my hand and told me that she needed to leave as her shift was over. This all happened right as I hit the transition stage, and in my emotional state I told her I wanted her to stay and begged her not to leave! She reassured me and said, "you're about to meet your baby!" I won't sugar-coat it; I found the transition period of labour difficult. I was sweating, felt nauseous, and there seemed to be no break in between contractions. I felt like I was losing control. I threw around some classic 'transition' statements such as, "I don't want to do this anymore", "I love this baby but I don't want to meet it today" and, "I want an epidural!" Despite all of this, it seemed to be over in seconds, and I remember the sweet relief of being able to push. It's hard to describe but pushing counteracted the intense pressure and almost neutralised the contractions. I can confirm (in my experience at least) that there definitely is a 'ring of fire', and it feels just like that; a ring of fire.

We laugh about it now, but someone repeatedly tried calling Jared, interrupting the music that was playing from his phone. The music was helping me focus, so I promptly asked for someone to, "get rid of that caller!" Olivia applied pressure to my perineum and coached me through my pushes. I still had the TENS machine going, although I don't think it was doing much other than proving a distraction for me by this stage.

At 5:08pm, my little baby joined us earth-side. It was magic. Jared announced, "It's a boy!" The room smelled warm. He was beautiful, and I felt like superwoman. I cried tears of joy, kissed him and marveled at the little human that I had grown and birthed. Delivery of the placenta was painless, and I don't even really remember it happening.

I had some grazing and a tear to the vaginal wall, curtesy of Eli trying to come out with his hand by his face! Olivia cleaned me up and Eli was able to do the breast crawl. We called family to announce Eli's birth, and to let my brother know that he correctly guessed Eli's sex, birth date and birth time within 20 minutes (he guessed 5:20pm!). An obstetrician rushed in stating that she needed to be quick as she was meant to be heading to theatre for another patient. She began assessing for perineal tears and I winced as everything felt so sensitive. She told me I needed some stitches and gave me a local anesthetic. I was adamant that I could still feel pain despite the anesthetic and asked her to stop. She told me, "you can't feel anything, it's numb". I felt so disregarded and scared and began to cry. Lovely Olivia stepped in and stopped the doctor, suggesting I could have stitches done in theatre. I was so thankful for Olivia in that moment. I agreed to go to theatre, and honestly, it was the best decision. I was relaxed and completely numb. Jared was able to stay with Eli for his weight and measurement checks and met me on the ward shortly after.

I still look back on my birth with fondness. I was supported, listened-to, respected and valued as an individual and as a mother.

Karyn and baby Eli

The birth of George

I'll give you a little background on myself, I was 18 when I found out I was expecting my first, a 'surprise' pregnancy! I was at university (training to be a nurse) so the timing was not great. I did some reading around birth, but to be honest most of my knowledge of birth came from TV shows, films, and the experience of older women around me (none of my friends had had children yet!). Also, being so young, I didn't ask any questions, I just did as I was told, and if I'm honest, I was terrified about the prospect of labour and birth! I think I also felt some embarrassment of being a 'teenage mum' and worried that care givers were judging me, so I didn't really talk about how I felt, I just wanted to be a 'good' patient.

When the day came I was actually very lucky, my son was born naturally and we were both well. However I ended up having diamorphine when I got to about 9cm as I felt completely out of control (I now know this is normal!). I only just got away with delivering without intervention after pushing for almost two hours.

My body was drained, although I only had first degree tearing, after two hours of pushing, everything swelled up to unrecognisable proportions. I was in a lot of pain postpartum. I don't have much family support (me and my mum don't speak and I have no sisters/cousins etc.) so it was just me and my partner, and we were clueless! I struggled my way through the postpartum period, tried to breastfeed but failed after a few weeks as I was in so much pain (with hindsight I now know my son was tongue tied) however no health professional picked up on this. Looking back I think I developed a degree of post-natal depression, but I didn't know at the time. It ended up being a very lonely and scary period of my life where I felt like I had no control over anything.

Second time around and 12 years later I became pregnant again. We left a big gap as me and my partner both needed to finish university and establish our careers. I am now 31 years old.

I knew that this time needed to different, I wanted this for both me and my baby. I didn't want to have opiates in labour, I wanted to breastfeed, I wanted to feel in control whilst bringing my baby into the world, and I didn't want to go through the feelings I experienced postpartum previously.

I had a difficult pregnancy this time around (my body was much better at growing a baby when I was younger!). I had lots of sickness, scans and tests, one minute I had too much fluid, the next I was having a huge baby, the next the baby had stopped growing, it was one thing after another. However, thanks to The Nurture Nest and The Hypnobirthing Podcast, and the knowledge I had gained I was able to stay calm, engage with the health care team around me, and make my own decisions.

My consultant wanted to induce me at 39 weeks due to the baby's growth slowing on what felt like my 100th scan. I did not want induction, the placental flow on the scan was fine, his movements were good and I felt like my body was naturally preparing for labour. After a long conversation with my consultant he admitted he didn't think anything was wrong, but because they had this piece of paper saying baby's growth had slowed he had to 'do' something. He also advised the measurements may not be completely accurate. Thanks to hypnobirthing I felt empowered to say no, I explained my decision that I did not want an induction. We compromised that I would return for another scan in one week, monitor baby's movements and have some sweeps in the meantime.

I had two sweeps over the next few days which didn't do much. I returned for my scan the following Wednesday and all was well with the placental flow. I was now 40 weeks and they gave me a third sweep whilst I was at the hospital and I agreed to induction on the Sunday (a full week and a half after they initially wanted to induce me). This sweep really got things moving, almost immediately. Unfortunately I went into a long drawn out latent labour with very strong contractions coming every 5 - 10 minutes. This went on from Wednesday to Sunday and without hypnobirthing I don't know how I would have coped. I remained calm and in control the whole time. With hindsight I don't know if I would accept sweeps again. I feel like my body would have laboured more effectively if I was left alone!

By the Saturday I was having such strong contractions that I wasn't sure if I could still feel baby moving properly so I went up to the hospital for a check, thankfully baby was fine but as I was due to be induced the next day, they kept me in for observation.

I was pretty sure I was in full blown labour by then, however no one examined me. In the morning the midwife came to tell me that there was no room on the labour ward and I would have to go home and come back tomorrow. I calmly explained again that I thought I was already in labour and I asked if someone could do a vaginal examination. Thanks to hypnobirthing I was again taking control of my care and doing what felt right for me and my baby.

A consultant came over and examined me. I was 6cm dilated and I was taken straight to the labour ward! My contractions remained strong but irregular for another few hours, but I now had gas and air which felt amazing after 5 days of labour with no pain relief! The midwife suggested artificially rupturing my membranes, and I agreed to this, again feeling totally in control as I understood the physiological process thanks to hypnobirthing. Two hours later I was holding my perfect baby boy in my hands. I gave birth on the floor (that is where I wanted to be) in the dark, with just gas and air. I let my body push my baby out, I breathed and constantly reminded myself that my body knew what to do. I barley had to push, I felt the fetal ejection reflex and I breathed and let it happen. I walked out of the delivery room 5 hours later to go home, not one tear or graze, a healthy baby in my arms and feeling like superwoman.

My feelings of happiness continued, as did my confidence. This time I was able to notice myself that my baby had tongue tie and couldn't latch and I arranged for an appointment for it to be snipped. I used hypnobirthing again to keep me calm when his latch felt like it was pulling my nipple off and through mastitis from engorgement as he couldn't empty my breast, and we got there in the end! We are happily breastfeeding 11 weeks down the line and he is a beautiful, content, calm baby.

Thank you Claire from the bottom of my heart for the amazing information you are putting out there which is actually changing lives. You do an amazing job and I hope you continue to promote hypnobirthing for many years to come! I will be taking some of the elements that I have learned from hypnobirthing and using it in my practice as a cancer nurse specialist to help my patients as it is such a valuable skill to have. It's changed my life and I wouldn't have known about it without your podcast. Thank you so much. Please keep up the amazing work that you are doing.

Myfanwy and baby George

The birth of Eddie

The day before I went into labour I had gone to the hospital with reduced movements as I hadn't felt the baby move much and was worried. Everything was fine and I was relieved when I left the hospital and felt much happier and my mind was put at ease. From the monitoring the midwife told me I was having braxton hicks but I couldn't really feel much. That evening my husband went to work for his night shift as normal and I had a bath and an early night.

I woke at 3am by my waters breaking 10 days before my due date, I felt so excited, I called my husband to let him know and said I was going to try and go back to sleep. I laid there for ages trying to sleep but I think I was too excited and it took over that I was finally going to meet my baby. I called the midwife at 5am as I had opted for a home birth to let them know. I then called my husband again and asked him to come home as my contractions had started.

The midwife came to us at 10:30am and timed my contractions and said she wasn't going anywhere and was staying. Everything was really calm and peaceful. In between contractions, we were chatting, making jokes and the midwife read some relaxations for me, we listened to a podcast, and I played my hypnobirthing music that I had been listening to throughout pregnancy. I had a bath at one point and it was so calming and through each contraction I practiced my breathing, the day just flew by!

At 6pm the pain started to increase and I was getting tired so I started the gas and air to help. The contractions where coming thick and fast and at about 8pm I requested to go to hospital as I wanted more pain relief. The midwife called for an ambulance but there was a 10 hour wait, I still wanted to go in so my husband drove me in. We arrived at the hospital at 9:10pm and I shut myself off from everyone. I went into my own zone using the down breathing technique and I stood holding a chair. The midwives asked me to go onto the bed but I told them I didn't want to lay down as standing was more comfortable for me. I kneeled on the bed and held onto the top of the bed and continued with the gas and air. When I got to the hospital my labour did not slow down I just focused and knew baby was close, I no longer wanted any other pain relief, something kicked in and I just wanted to get him here safely. I certainly didn't breathe my baby out and I was not as calm as earlier in the day, but I just did what was comfortable to me. I listened to the midwives and with their help Eddie was born at 10:14pm. The midwife gave him a little rub and laid him on my chest and we had delayed cord clamping.

If I had known before I left home how soon Eddie would have been here I am sure I would have stayed at home. But it was a blessing as we stayed in hospital for 2 nights, my husband was able to stay too and we had support with breastfeeding and a midwife with me every time I fed Eddie to help him latch on. I wouldn't have got this being at home so it all worked out well for a reason.

The only negative of going to hospital was I felt like we didn't get that hour after birth of just the three of us, there seemed to be something going on constantly after the birth when I just wanted to just cuddle my baby with my husband. Only a few minutes after birth they asked if I wanted an injection for the placenta, I declined and said can we give it 10 minutes to see if this happens naturally, two minutes later the placenta came on its own while I held onto Eddie.

Although my birth didn't exactly go to plan, I did just panic and suddenly wanted to be in hospital however, my birth experience is very positive and I love sharing it and letting people know that it can be positive. Others were desperate to tell me their horror stories and I just blocked this out. I was very positive in the lead up to my labour and I believe this was down to hypnobirthing. I listened to podcasts, read books, practiced my breathing and listening to my relaxation music every day; it all helped build my confidence.

I wouldn't change anything about my labour. After a few days of having Eddie me and my husband were talking of having another baby because it was such an amazing experience I can't wait to do it all again!

Pippa and baby Eddie

The birth of Shalev

As soon as I found out I was pregnant I was determined to prepare for birth, like you would for any other momentous and potentially challenging event. The focus was on learning the physiology as much as possible rather than what colour to paint the nursery walls! (I left that to my husband). I didn't want an unnecessary traumatic event in my life.

I listened to hypnobirthing audiobooks and MP3s most days, the affirmations became very comforting and I would often fall asleep to the guided meditations. Another amazing source of information was The Hypnobirthing Podcast, in particular the Kemi Johnson episode.

It really started to open my eyes to the conveyor belt of interventions that maternity services put forward. As I was not aware on the effects of induction on intervention rates. My best friend also had a traumatic first birth and warned me against accepting any pethidine straight away! "Just undermines the belief in yourself".

I really listened to experienced friends who have birthed. My best/most common question was, "how do you know when to push?" They all reassured me I would know and so did the resources above. The urge to push into my bottom did come after 1.5 hours and I sure did.

It took nearly 3 years to conceive baby Shalev, and subsequently it only happened through NHS IUI after a very early pregnancy loss. We are very thankful for the NHS fertility services and help we received. We were very lucky to get free fertility treatment during Covid.

My pregnancy was a dream including no sickness. I was relaxed throughout and stayed active. I completed NHS breastfeeding classes with the hospital, antenatal and free online courses, including yoga and relaxation. As recommended by the hospital I started colostrum harvesting at 38 weeks which I believe definitely brought on the labour and increased my oxytocin.

My hospital had set my induction "date" by saying I couldn't go to the birth centre if I went over 42 weeks. So I needed to be induced on 8th December at 41 + 4 days.

Even though my 12 week scan put me 4 days ahead of my IUI date and date of last period! Which is crazy as we knew exactly when he was conceived. I was not that big or uncomfortable and definitely could carry this baby beyond 42 weeks! I had also measured small twice and been given extra scans, but I was confident this baby was fine and he would end up being about 7 to 7.5lbs. Correct final weight 7lbs 2oz.

So here goes: on Sunday 28th November - the 1st night of Hanukkah I noticed I lost a bit of liquid (but just assumed it was wee or discharge!)

The next morning I saw it again but still the penny didn't drop. After walking the dog with a family friend, I mentioned the drip and she said the same thing happened with her 2nd child exactly 32 years previously and to get it checked out.

Once home and after eating a large lunch including cookie dough and ice cream, a bit more liquid emerged. I phoned triage and they said to come in urgently if waters had broken because of the risk of infection with no contractions. Plus I was approaching the 24 hours mark. I was told a syntocinon IV would start at 6pm on the labour ward. And it would be "rapid with no respite as this baby must be born ASAP due to risk of infection".

Due to my hypnobirthing I was calm and happy; labour had started naturally so my hormones levels must be at the right levels. As we drove home my husband picked up his prescription and I had a light surge in the car.

Once home I noticed my bloody show and my contractions started properly. I was in my comfortable safe space and the need to empty my bowels started. I continued walking around the house breathing 4 in 8 out. Plus the affirmations naturally sprung into mind. At this point I thought I best record the surges. I recorded 7 surges within 20 minutes all over a minute each.

I still was not in a rush to get back to the hospital and we stopped at the shop for Hairbo. At this point I could not record my surges and just had to focus on the affirmations and breathing. Heading down the A10 it continued to gather intensity with only 30 second rest break between each one.

Even though I have worked at my hospital for 7 years I have never driven to the maternity part of the hospital. So we drove around a few times! Before sneaking through the loading bay entrance.

My husband dropped me off and I had another surge in the toilet. Once in triage they said they would start the drip shortly. I explained I didn't think it was necessary!

Then I was taken to the birth centre for an assessment. The two on duty midwifes straight away put me ease and calmed the situation and allowed me space, they followed the ethos of hypnobirthing.

They offered me pain relief -my first response was no as my friend had told me the out on control feeling of pethidine. I needed to know where things were at. I wanted to stay in control. They then offered me gas and air. My husband encouraged me to have it, it was something I was familiar with already. And as soon as I inhaled that I knew I could use it to regulate my breathing even further. I knew I could do this and it would really take the edge off. I remember seeing the midwifes hand come out of my vagina looking really open but I told myself likely to be 2 or 3 cm dilated best case scenario. But she looked at me and said "about 9cms" very calmly. Having read and understood the different stages of labour I knew I was heading in the right direction and knew with confidence I can do this!

Due to the infection risk I still needed IV antibiotics via my hand - oral not an option. This was annoying and took several attempts to connect as surges were coming quick.

We moved room again and I clung to the gas and air. I positioned myself on the bed on all fours and remembered the birthing positions I had learnt. Using gravity was all I could think. Within minutes of being in that room I felt the need to push just like described by my female friends. With each surge I pushed into my bottom as much as possible. I was really focused on letting my friend in New Zealand know that I was in labour so between contractions we FaceTimed and that was when I got a bit emotional and she told me give it my all. The pushing stage was about 1.5 hours, and beside me was my husband telling me to channel into the push rather than yell, (although I think he was repeating what the midwife said).

The midwives changed at 8pm and I was worried I'd lose my momentum but I stayed focused. I remembered sometimes you can have a wobble at this point, and keeping with hypnobirthing I didn't ask what point I was at. I just stayed with my body and listened to what it was telling me to do. Once I felt the ring of fire I knew it was getting closer, it kind of felt good. The midwife tried to guide me to push slowly to avoid tearing but to be honest the sensation was more manageable. A vagina is definitely designed for this to occur and I wasn't really bothered about tearing.

I'm pleased my husband also didn't really let me know where things were at and stayed beside me helping with the breathing control. I remember my friend telling me you will feel the imprint of his face. Within seconds I felt the swish of his body through me. It was amazing and I knew straight away he was fine. A deep purple colour.

We were not even as emotional as I thought we would be. We both just felt relieved and just so happy to have Shalev here. Passing the placenta was more boring than anything else. By that time I was too preoccupied with his skin to skin to the notice anything. My husband cut the cord, I am rhesus negative so delaying the cord clamp was not really an option.

I had a bit of gas here for the stitches and started expressing and giving Shalev colostrum immediately. Without doing all this preparation I know I would not have been in a position to be confident and could've got scared at any point. I hope more woman have faith in their bodies and are allowed to have an amazing experience. We seem to be in conflict a little with some aspects of the maternity services. I am so thankful for how well everything went and how I was able to then concentrate fully on being a new Mum and establish breastfeeding.

I feel like I've given my son and myself the best start possible and just wanted to share it with anyone who will listen, I'm so proud of myself.

Hypnobirthing has given me the best start to motherhood beyond just the birth. I am so thankful for all the preparation, a lot of friends say I was lucky but I know it was being educated and knowledgeable that allowed us to have this positive story. I highly recommend expecting mothers to take time to prepare and educate themselves for this experience as I feel knowledge is key and has been the reason for this positive experience

Robyn and baby Shalev

The birth of Hope

Hope was due 7th November 2019 and we had planned for a water birth at our local birth centre in Maidstone, Kent. In preparation we had taken a hypnobirthing course at the birth centre which was taught by a midwife, Shona, who worked there. We found the course super helpful and felt prepared for however the birth unfolded.

On the due date I was just relaxing at home and I remember calling my Dad during the morning and saying that my bump felt tighter than usual and maybe something was happening. By lunchtime I could still feel the tightening and I felt like it was more difficult to feel the baby move. Just to check everything was okay we called our local hospital who invited us to come in that afternoon for monitoring. As it was my due date we took our hospital bags in case this was it! We were seen quickly at the hospital and the heart monitor confirmed baby was doing fine and I was starting to have mild contractions. After the monitoring the midwife asked if I wanted to be examined as I had mentioned I thought my mucus plug had gone during the night. I was expecting the midwife to advise that it would still be a while yet and my cervix was still closed, however, to my surprise she said I was 2cm dilated and I was so happy to hear this. I felt that I'd achieved those 2cm without really knowing that things were underway. We left the hospital and drove home, picking up dinner on the way. I was uncomfortable in the car as the contractions had started to pick up. At home I got myself comfy lying on the bed with a pregnancy pillow, TENS machine, essential oils and my hypnobirthing tracks whilst my partner cooked us dinner.

The contractions continued fairly regularly although I didn't time them and they were manageable using the TENS machine and breathing techniques I'd learned through hypnobirthing. After dinner, we settled on the sofa to watch TV and around 8pm the contractions stopped. I was mildly relieved as I was getting tired and increasingly uncomfortable but also disappointed that this might not be it just yet. I went to bed and got a full nights rest (with the exception of a few wee breaks). The next morning my contractions restarted at around 8:30am. I got my partner to put the TENS machine on and I tried to relax and watch a film (Bad Moms Xmas) however unlike the previous night these contractions were increasingly intense and I started to doubt whether I could breathe my way through them. I continued to labour at home until around 10am when after a contraction I felt my water break. At this point we decided to call our local birthing centre, they asked a few questions and invited us to come in to see how I was getting on. I was pleased to be heading in and really didn't want them to send me back home again as I knew I would feel more comfortable at the birth centre. We arrived and were shown into one of the birthing suites and I was so pleased that the midwife who came to examine me was Shona who'd taught our hypnobirthing classes. At that moment I was relieved to see a familiar face. Whilst I was being examined my waters then fully burst and the midwife explained that I was around 6cms dilated however due to there being meconium in the waters we would need to be transferred to our local hospital. This was so the baby could be closely monitored as the meconium could be a sign the baby was in distress. We knew that transferring to the hospital was a possibility as this had been explained to us during a previous visit to the birth centre. It was very calm and relaxing whilst we waited for an ambulance and I was soon on my way with the paramedics and my partner Dom followed behind in the car. Labouring in the ambulance wasn't easy as I was strapped to the gurney for safety. I used the gas and air to help breathe through each contraction and began to wonder whether I should ask for an epidural once I reached the hospital.

Once we arrived at the delivery suite I was settled into a room by a midwife (I think her name was Lottie) she attached a monitor onto the baby's head and also checked my progress. The ambulance ride had certainly sped things up as I was now 9cms dilated and so I thought well I've come this far on gas and air, I can do this, baby is almost here. By now it was around 12:30pm. I continued to labour on the bed switching between laying on my back and being on my knees facing the back of the bed which I found the most comfortable. After another hour I was fully dilated and ready to begin pushing. I was still most comfortable on my knees however baby didn't agree and her heart rate was dipping slighting after each push/contraction and taking longer to recover than the midwife would have liked. The midwife took the decision at this stage to push the emergency buzzer for extra help. The room filled with doctors and nurses who all remained calm and explained that we needed to get baby out soon. I moved onto my back as this position was better for baby's heart rate and I pushed with all I had and although I was making progress it was 2 steps forward 1 step back and so I was offered an episiotomy which I agreed to. Shortly after this and several more pushes baby Hope was born. After an initial quick check over due to the meconium in her waters we had our first cuddle and breastfeed. Hope then had some skin-on-skin time with Dom whilst I had my stitches and my favoured part of giving birth; a cup of tea and some toast! We stayed at the hospital overnight as Hope needed to be monitored every 2 hours. Her stats were always fine and the meconium had not caused any issues. We headed home the following afternoon to begin our lives as a family of 3.

Debbie and baby Hope

INDUCTION BIRTH

The birth of Mila

      Living abroad can present a multitude of challenges that we have to learn to navigate. My husband plays professional hockey in Europe, so we are currently living in Northern Italy. When we became pregnant back in April, I knew I wanted to mentally and physically prepare for a natural birth since we would be somewhere in Europe, where labor seemed less medicalized than back home in North America. I did not want to go in expecting pain medication, only to not have received them; I feel that would send me into a panic. So preparing for a natural birth as best I could seemed like good homework for the next 9 months.

      My friend introduced me to hypnobirthing, which I dove into on our 10 hour flight overseas. I came across The Hypnobirthing Podcast, and started binging each episode. My husband and I decided to sign up for Claire's group classes, as we wanted to feel confident and informed about the labor and delivery process. Over the next few months, I practiced breathing techniques, researched what was available to me here in Italy, and prepared a birth preference plan that I could go over with the midwife. Here in Italy, I was faced with a language barrier, so I wanted to try and be informed and confident so I could properly advocate for myself, since my husband was not allowed at the appointments due to COVID (he speaks Italian, but they still wouldn't let him come in as my translator).

      My last appointment was at 37 weeks, and everything looked good. Baby girl was in a great position, and it felt like she could come any day because she was low.

During week 38, I kept experiencing a *very* small amount of liquid leaking. Pee? Discharge? Amniotic fluid? The three liquids it could possibly be. Everything I looked up said that if it was amniotic fluid, it would continue leaking. Mine wasn't. It would be a small amount one day, then nothing for days, then another small amount another day. So I ignored it.

Week 39, I started to panic a bit because she was so active, I could have sworn she did a flip and put herself in a breech position. Because of my anterior placenta, it was difficult to map her. I decided to go into the hospital just to check; for peace of mind. Upon monitoring me, they noticed my amniotic fluid was low. They tested me, but the result came back negative. The doctor told me she was confused as to why my fluid was so low, but the test was negative. They told me that if I leaked ANYTHING, that I needed to come back to the hospital to check if it was amniotic fluid right away. Not being able to fully communicate with the midwife and doctor, it was hard to tell how urgent this was. This all had me feeling very uneasy. The next day, I sat around my apartment afraid to move, and constantly monitoring my body. Mentally, it put me in a bad spot. The next day, I felt something leak. My husband was so amazing, and taking what he learned from the course about being a strong support, he knew exactly what I needed. We headed to the hospital, if anything, for peace of mind.

Another negative test result for amniotic fluid. After an ultrasound, the doctor told me that I had plenty of amniotic fluid and that I shouldn't be concerned at all and should go on living life normally. The conflicting information from two visits, only a day apart, had my head spinning. But I needed to get back into a positive head space, because her due date was 6 days away. I was able to wash away the worry with meditation and affirmations, getting my mind and body reconnected.

On Christmas day, we headed up the mountain for a lunch with our hockey family. I started to feel some discomfort, but attributed it to Braxton Hicks. I was, after all, only 3 days away. Once we returned home and got ready for the night, I noticed some leaking. I immediately thought it was amniotic fluid, but it wasn't a constant leak...I wanted to trust my gut, but I kept having the doctors voice in my head and the negative test result. So I went to bed. As I lay there I felt another leak, but this time it was more. I felt that this was it. I was leaking amniotic fluid, and we needed to head to the hospital.

We got our baby bag and headed to the hospital around 11pm Christmas night. We were both so calm and felt so ready for whatever. From my research, I knew that I might have to be induced if she didn't come naturally, but I wasn't sad or mad about the possibility of a sudden change to our birth preferences. I felt totally calm.

Once we arrived at the hospital, I buzzed for the midwife. I went back for monitoring and testing, while my husband waited in the lobby. Once the door closed, I quickly realized that I had a midwife who spoke zero English. The panic began to set in, as I didn't know how we'd communicate efficiently enough. Because she couldn't speak to me, she somewhat just went about what their protocol would be for checking for amniotic fluid. Fear and discomfort began to set in as she performed a pelvic exam without consent (I thought it was going to be a test for amniotic fluid). I immediately felt violated and angry, especially since my husband, who she could communicate with, was right outside the door. Once she removed her fingers, fluid gushed out. I then knew my membrane had ruptured, but it must have been a very tiny leak, resulting in a small amount of fluid loss over the past few weeks. She performed a test, and it came back positive this time. Without saying anything else, she looked at me and said,

"You stay," and left the room. I took that as a 'you have to stay at the hospital tonight' but, again, wasn't 100% sure. She left me for an hour, hooked up to a monitor, pondering what was going to happen. Listening to the beep of my baby's heart beat kept me calm, and I did my best to breathe and reassure myself that all will be okay. Our baby would be okay. I would be okay.

As I continued to lay there though, the frustration set in. I begged the midwife to let me see my husband so I could talk to him. He plays such an important role in the delivery of our baby, as my partner and support. He's the one who can keep me calm and can advocate for me and knows what I want and do not want. But they were taking that away from me. Eventually, through tears and anger, I demanded he be let in, and they finally agreed.

He was such a calm presence, when he could have been very angry, especially with how things were going so far. After he talked with the midwife, he relayed the message that I would have to stay the night at the hospital, be given an antibiotic drip, and hope that my body begins to go into labor naturally. I was going to be given a new drip every 6 hours, and hooked up to the monitor every 4 hours. If nothing happened by 1PM the following day, they were going to induce me.

Now that my husband and I had worked together to reestablish my *calm*, we said our goodbye's and I headed to my room to rest. I felt a very strong connection to my baby and my body, and I knew she was not going to kick start the labor process. So I mentally prepared to be induced and did my research on inductions as I laid in bed. Because an induction is forcing your body into labor, I knew the contractions were going to be way more intense (confirmed by the nurses and midwife the next day), so I also researched what medications might be offered for pain, and calmly accepted the fact that my natural, unmedicated water birth was most likely going to become an induced, medicated, bed delivery. And I was okay, because my baby was okay. I also listened to the positive induction story from the podcast and felt so reassured that my body was not failing me, and that this was just how it was going to be. No matter what, the safe delivery of my baby is what mattered the most.

The next day, at 1pm, I saw the doctor. She did not speak English. The midwife did not speak English. Panic set in as they tried to explain how they were going to insert something into me and monitor me another 24 hours. I was so confused because I had never heard, read, or seen anything about this tampon they were showing me. But they couldn't explain to me what it was. I told them that they were absolutely NOT going to be inserting ANYTHING into me without me knowing what it was. Irritated, they asked me to call my husband so he could translate. My husband relayed that it was a tampon/string soaked in prostaglandins what will, hopefully, kick start contractions over the next 24 hours. There was also the option of taking a pill of prostaglandins every 4 hours until contractions began, but they didn't want me to take that option because they wanted me to sleep through the night and get some rest without being woken up to take a pill. These were two options I did not read about. Luckily, a midwife that spoke English (Claudia) clocked on, and she came and spoke with me and was so calm and wonderful. After being able to ask the risks and benefits of each option, I felt confident in the doctor's decision to use this method of induction. If it wasn't for the hypnobirthing class, I'm not sure I would have had the confidence to advocate for myself in a room full of people who couldn't understand me - I might have just gone along with whatever they said, uncomfortable as it may have made me.

Around midnight I began to feel the surges. They were very mild, and I felt so excited and ready to begin the process of bringing our baby girl into this world. There wasn't an ounce of fear in my body. I welcomed each surge, and fell back asleep knowing it was going to be a big day for the Bardaro family. At 2am, the surges became much more intense. They were regular and ramping up in intensity over the hours. I used my breathing to get through each one. I did my best to remain active, pausing when needed to breathe through the surges. Around 5:30am, I knew it was time to slowly waddle my way to the delivery side, and I called my husband to come to the hospital.

They hooked me up to the monitor and could see that my contractions were very intense already. An English-speaking midwife was on duty, so communicating was finally easy. I let them know my husband was in the lobby, and they said he couldn't come in yet until I was dilated more. I remained extremely firm in my request for him to be present, especially since a different doctor and midwife had told me he can be with me as soon as I went to the delivery side. So much conflicting information! They agreed to let my husband in. They let us know that, although my contractions were very intense, they were not doing much, as I was only 1cm dilated. I asked when I could receive the epidural, and they said at 5cm. We left the observation room and went to a delivery room. We kept the room dark, and I laid on the bed, eyes closed, breathing through each surge with my husband's reassuring voice at my side. My midwife (Maddalena) was so sweet and such a calming presence. The next few hours went by peacefully.

Around 3cm dilated, things really ramped up. Each surge was so intense. I requested to use the shower, which was in a different part of the delivery ward. The hot water helped so much! Although I was unable to labor in the birth tub, I was very happy to utilize some form of water, as it's an extreme comfort to me. Because of the pain, I begged my midwife for something to take the edge off. At that point, I knew I couldn't continue without something to help alleviate the intensity of each surge. The midwife agreed, so we made our way back to the delivery room. They administered a mild opioid drip—honestly, I'm not 100% sure what I was given. I was in my own world at that point, trying to get through each surge. My husband spoke for me. Whatever it was, it worked for about an hour, which was a nice reset. I was able to really relax between the contractions and finally drink some electrolytes, which I needed. I also demanded that my husband go down to the cafeteria to get something to eat, as it had been hours since he ate anything, and I was okay on my own, in my head, breathing and connecting with my baby.

By the time he returned (about 20-30 minutes), I reached 5cm. They called for the anesthesiologist. It took 30-45 minutes for him to arrive. In that time, I went from 5cm to 9cm. Those surges were taking me past my pain threshold, but with the help and encouragement from my husband and midwife, I got through them. I moved to a different delivery room. Hunched over on the bed, waiting for the needle, I felt an urge to push. Fluid gushed out. I couldn't move, though. They informed me that, because I was 9cm dilated, they couldn't administer a full epidural because they wanted me to feel pushing and be able to walk. Honestly, I thought the purpose of an epidural was to NOT feel anything, but I trusted my midwife and knew she wouldn't do something to further my discomfort.

After I received the epidural, my midwife informed me that I was 10cm dilated, and that if I felt the urge to push, to go ahead. My epidural did not take, and I pushed for 2.5 hours. I was so exhausted, each push draining me more and more. The left side of my cervix was blocking the head a bit, so with consent, my midwife gently helped to moved it so I could continue pushing. We tried multiple positions. I felt like my baby wasn't helping me much, and I tried so hard to connect with her and encourage her out. "I can see her hair!

She's right there!" Those words coming from my husband gave me such reassurance! The midwife told me to reach down and feel her head. In doing so, I became so motivated and got a huge rush of energy. I knew I was going to meet her soon. I kept repeating my affirmation in my head, "I will meet my baby soon. I will meet my baby soon." I had to change positions to my knees, as I knew she needed gravity for assistance. A few pushes later, and her head came out. Words of encouragement filled the room as I gave a few more pushes during the last contractions. "Reach down and catch your baby!" I let go of the back of the bed and reached down to catch my daughter as she entered the world. Truly the most incredible experience I have ever had. I completely forgot about the pain and discomforts labor brought on. I was overwhelmed with happiness and pride. I pulled her up to my chest and held her. She laid there, alert and so peaceful. We did it, baby girl!

Mila Lyne Bardaro came into this world at 4:57pm on December 27th, 2021 weighing 7lbs 5oz, 20 inches long. She is perfection, and we could not be more in love.

Chelsea and baby Mila

The birth of Molly

I am a 32 year old healthy women, although was looking forward to having a baby I had no idea what pregnancy and birthing would be like.

The 12-week scan was the first time I realised that in order to have a baby I would need to have a birth. I immediately enrolled upon a hypnobirthing course. I had no clue what birth entailed and had heard some terrible accounts of what could be coming my way.

Hypnobirthing taught us a huge amount. We were fascinated to learn that there was so much to a woman's body that we never knew existed. We watched birth videos and read birth stories as well as listening to podcasts and positive birth stories. Each morning on the way to work I listened to the birth affirmations and politely told others that I didn't want to know what had happened at their birth. My most important affirmation was "I am a strong."

Throughout the pregnancy I slowly became less scared and more excited for the birth. We had written down our birth preferences and knew what we wanted- as much time at home before active labour, to birth in the midwife led unit, a vaginal birth into water, and as little pain relief as possible. I really didn't want medical intervention and was sure that there was no need for this to happen.

Despite a sickly start to the pregnancy everything was going well, we had the birth plan written and the bags packed. We knew the route to the hospital, and I had endless snacks parceled up and a set of baby clothes ready for our new arrival. I had booked a series of acupuncture sessions from 38 weeks to support a natural birth.

It was all going to plan until the 38 week appointment when the midwife put the paper tape measure on my tummy and said that the baby's growth had reduced. She advised we went to the hospital and had a growth scan that day. Just a little hiccup we thought.

The sonographer and her student both checked over my bump and seemed happy enough, they even said we had a very active baby who was head down and snuggled up nicely ready to be born. We sat in the hospital waiting room and were all ready to go home and wait a few more weeks until labour began.

Soon after we were invited in to speak to the midwife, and this is when things began to change. The midwife told us that the growth of the baby had decreased. The measurements they had taken of the baby's body were reduced and there was a chance that the placenta was beginning to fail, this could affect the baby's development and growth. The consultant and midwife suggested induction. This was not in the birth plan.

At this point I began to crumble and explained politely to the midwife that induction wasn't in my birth plan. Thanks, but no thanks.

Luckily my husband Joe stepped in and was able ask lots of sensible questions whilst I gathered myself together - I had totally forgotten BRAINS and was staring into space imagining a birth pool being drained and the birthing plan now a paper airplane flying out the window.

The midwife was wonderful, she talked us through all the details, the benefits, risks, alternatives. After this chat I felt much better. Given the medical advice and the circumstances we decided that we would book to be induced 72 hours later. After a long conversation with midwives and consultants, induction seemed the safest thing to do for our baby.

We asked if I could be examined and if I could be given a sweep every day until I was to go in to be induced as this may encourage labour to start naturally.

Over the next 72 hours we did lots to get ready. We knew oxytocin would help bring on labour, so we did everything. I had induction acupuncture, went on long walks, visited our favourite places, laughed, ate amazing foods, I harvested some colostrum ready for our little one, we talked about our new baby, had a big curry and drank raspberry leaf tea and generally tried to relax. We listened to our hypnobirthing tracks and affirmation to go to sleep and read the affirmations as we had throughout pregnancy.

I had three sweeps in total and each time we visited the midwife at the hospital we asked more questions. This allowed us to feel increasingly informed and reassured.

We genuinely felt it was our decision and there was no pressure to follow the less "natural route". We wanted a safe and beautiful delivery, and this is what the hospital team wanted too.

Sunday came around and natural labour had not begun, we checked in at the hospital later in the afternoon and they began monitoring the baby. Unfortunately, as we were due to be induced, we couldn't be in the midwife led unit and needed to be in consultant led care. The upside it turns out was we had our own room and bathroom and my husband could stay the whole time. The monitoring began and due to a very busy hospital ward mid-pandemic it wasn't until 2am on Monday that the consultant came round to start the first stage of the induction.

The first stage was to have a pessary fitted, this would be in place for 24 hours and the idea was that this would help prepare the cervix and allow contractions to begin.

It was a long 24 hours of being upright, active and forward and to cut a long day short nothing changed, I had some mild period pains but nothing that felt like a baby arriving.

Cut to Tuesday 2am and the midwife examined me, removed the pessary and said that the pessary had encouraged me to dilate to 1cm, she felt my cervix and described it as "favourable", and they then recommended I had my waters broken as they felt that this would encourage natural contractions.

I was not too sure and so we asked if we could have a break in the induction and wait to see if these mild period pains were the start of natural labour. After a nap and some chocolate nothing happened. Six hours later we were no further. I was quite tired and starting to wonder how long this would take.

This is when the most wonderful midwife came onto shift, her name was Bec and she was a breath of fresh air. She listened to us; we told her the birth plan had gone out the window, I had a little cry.

She totally understood and told us the birth plan was not out the window and was still relevant. She suggested that the consultant came and chatted to us to and reassure us. The consultant and midwife came back and were both incredible women, they were both hugely knowledgeable about hypnobirthing and were keen for me to have a natural birth. The consultant told me she had had two babies and delivered them both naturally following induction – this was just the positivity I needed.

We decided that having my waters broken was the right thing to do, we wanted our baby here safely and this would bring her here closer.

At 12pm Bec and the consultant broke my waters, they chatted to me about my job and somehow made breaking waters seem like the exciting start to meeting our baby. It didn't seem invasive, and they were so calm. I listened to my relaxation tracks and visualised birthing.

There was a trickle of water on the bed, and it began. Within the hour I was feeling something happen. I was marching around the room stretching and leaning on all the surfaces. All the birthing positions we had practiced suddenly came to me from nowhere, I instinctively moved into lots of positions and my husband offered me food, water and a back massage. The sensations I was experiencing came and went and I began counting my breaths.

For some reason, I visualised a clock. I had never done it before, but I was breathing through the contractions in clockwise rotations whilst imagining a hand tick round a clock, 5 seconds inhale, and 5 out.

For me the contractions felt like strong period cramps. I could manage each one but it all happened quickly I was not sure how long I could keep going for as it was very exhausting. The midwife came in and checked on me and asked me how I was doing. After two hours there wasn't much gap between the contractions, and I had a wobble. I wasn't sure that I could do it - in my mind labour was going to be at least 12 hours and this was only the first couple. I had never considered labour in a hospital may happen quickly. It was quite scary thinking I would have to do this for a long time.

Joe was a wonderful advocate, he talked to the midwives so I didn't need to. He was the voice of reason and explained to the midwife that I had really wanted a water birth and if the delivery room with a pool was available, we would like to use the wireless monitoring system to have our baby. I didn't think there was much chance of this but it's always worth asking.

We were moved through to the delivery suite after an hour or so - time seemed like a blur for me. I couldn't keep track; Joe had all that covered so I just did my thing.

The delivery suite was amazing; dimmed lights, calming music, lots of space and had a huge pool in it. I was over the moon. I was introduced to a wonderful midwife Phoebe and her student Emily. They were so relaxed and truly wonderful people.

I was finding it tough and asked the midwife if I could have further pain relief. The midwife held my birth plan in her hand and said "Lucy I've read your plan, I don't think you want pain relief" I'll remember this forever - the birth plan was relevant, it was worth doing, it had a place! I was a strong woman, and I knew I could do it and having the support of everyone was wonderful.

The midwife examined me as my contractions were thick and fast. To her surprise I had gone from 1cm dilated to 9cm. She later told me that at this examination she had expected me to be 3cm dilated!

The student midwife Emily was tasked with filling the pool. Not an easy job under pressure on your first day of midwife placement it turns out!

I moved around the room freely and being monitored wirelessly. For some unknown reason I felt the need to begin doing squats! No, I have never wanted to do squats before or since, but it turns out in labour this felt great!

Gas and air is also a wonderful thing, I used my breathing techniques to help me do big long breaths of gas and air. After 9 months of no alcohol, this was quite a lovely feeling. It helped me breathe and it helped me focus on the baby.

I began to feel the baby coming and to my surprise felt I wanted to push, this was the most comfortable part of the birth, the contractions felt purposeful, and every feeling made me know our baby was coming. The pool was ready just in time. As I got into the pool the relief was unbelievable. I felt like I was floating and every muscle in my body took a sigh. The water was warm and moved around my body beautifully. I knew I needed to push, no one told me this would happen so soon but something inside made me know I was ready. I was not scared I was not in pain; my body was doing it.

The midwife put a mirror on the floor of the pool, and I squatted in the pool facing Joe who held me. It was intense, but it was so natural. I was not hurting or scared I was just having a baby and somehow the world stopped turning and I just went with it.

Holding my husband's hands and being surrounded by amazing midwives my little girl was being born. Within a minute I had birthed the head, I felt my little girls head as she appeared into the water. I was so proud of her already and with one more push she was here. The midwife passed her between my legs, and I held her. She took a little minute to realise she was here and then let out a huge cheer to let us know she was here.

The emotion and feeling were incredible I was so proud of us both and of this bundle of baby.

Our little girl, Molly, was born at 39 weeks weighing 6lbs 12oz and she is wonderful.

I was in active labour for 2 hours and 25 minutes. It was the most intense and powerful experience of my life and one I would not change in any way.

We set out thinking induction was not for us, but it was the perfect birth for us on the day.

The NHS staff are remarkable people, and I cannot thank them enough for being wonderful professionals but also amazing humans.

Lucy and baby Molly

The birth of Aurelia

I am over the moon to be sharing my birth story and I really hope that somebody who is following hypnobirthing can read this and it will be some help, comfort and support for them.

First trimester I very much struggled with morning sickness but aside from that up until 36 weeks I very much had a text book pregnancy. I do love pregnancy and I think it is a real honour to be growing another human. After all the research I had done into hypnobirthing I had decided that I wanted a home birth and this was going to give me the birthing experience that I so wanted. I was awaiting my 36 week appointment with the midwife to know that everything was looking well with the baby and then I was going to book my pool.

When I attended my 36 week midwife appointment the midwife discovered that the baby was transverse. At this stage I didn't know a great deal of what having a transverse baby meant and I went for a scan that day with an open mind. When I arrived for the scan the baby had turned to frank breech which meant my babies bum was at the exit and legs were by the baby's head. We were given four options at this stage. To do nothing, book for an ECV, prepare for a breech delivery or to book a caesarean. Using the BRAIN model we decided we wanted to try an ECV.

We were booked in for an ECV 4 days later. I decided to wait to order my pool until we knew the outcome of the ECV. I won't lie, the 4 days waiting was tough and I did a lot of research and tried to block out any negativity people had around ECV's as it was my decision to opt for this.

We arrived for the ECV and the consultant scanned me and I was over the moon to discover that now my baby was head down. I went home and booked our pool for home.

My 38 week appointment with the midwife came and the baby was back transverse. We opted to have a scan the next day to give the baby time to move. This time the baby was footling breech which means the baby's feet were below its bottom. We saw the consultant after the scan and he wanted to admit me there and then to get booked in for a caesarean in the next few days. I asked to go home, the consultant explained the risk of cord prolapse to me if my waters were to break but both of my previous pregnancies went to 41+ weeks so I felt at 38 weeks the likelihood was this baby wasn't coming yet. I asked for a second opinion of what my options were and we would discuss them the next day. That night I was searching everybody's caesarean stories to get my head around that this was likely going to be our birth outcome. It really was helpful for me to discover how I could still make it my birth while it not being my preferred option. The next day the consultant rang and agreed for me to wait another week and come back to be rescanned. I did so much research, I extended my birth preferences to ensure they included every outcome as previously I had tried not to look at caesareans, forceps etc. because this was not what I wanted.

39 weeks came and I was rescanned and the baby was head down and I was sent home. I was hugely relieved and was excited that we were back on track.

A few days later I was certain the baby had flipped again so we went back in. The scan did show that the baby was head down but because now it was classed as an unstable lie they wanted me in for an induction. I discussed my options with them and again used the BRAIN model. I chose that I was happy with an induction and a vaginal delivery was really important to me and I knew how upset I would have been if the baby did flip again and it resulted in a caesarean.

I had the pessary inserted at 11am, unfortunately at our hospital with induction you do need to stay in once they have begun the process but I was adamant I would not be strapped to a hospital bed. We walked round the hospital the whole day until I had to go back to be monitored 6 hours later. My partner and I did 12500 steps that day! My partner was sent home at 9pm and I was put back on the monitor at 12.30am. I could feel very slight tightening's and did wonder if these would develop. I put my head phones in and fell asleep watching Friends.

My partner came back at 8am, I was examined at 12.30pm and the decision was to insert the first 6 hour gel. We had been moved to a private room at this point but were not in a room with a pool and we had consistently informed them that I was wanting a water birth. I knew if I went on the hormone drip that it would be unlikely I'd be able to have a water birth. I did feel at this stage the midwife wasn't pushing for me to have the water birth but I left it at this stage as I still wasn't in labour and knew it could be a while longer, so off we went walking. I was getting more regular tightening's but I was talking, laughing, walking through them. I had downloaded the Freya app but didn't want to time anything as I wanted to leave my mind clear and I felt as I was already at hospital I didn't need to time them as nothing was dependent on how close they were together or how long they were lasting. My partner had noticed while we were out walking that the frequency had definitely increased but I reassured him that had we been at home we would still would not be ringing the hospital yet.

We went back to our room about 5pm and I bounced on the ball and watched Friends (we had discussed this would keep my oxytocin levels up) I was starting to have to close my eyes through the surges and began counting my up breathing. I was doing ok and my focus was on getting to 7pm as I knew I was going to be checked at that stage and I could make a plan of how I was doing with the surges. 7pm came and a student midwife popped her head in and just asked how I was doing and left. This is when I had a little wobble. I switched to the hypnobirthing MP3's as I could feel myself getting near to the red zone during surges and I needed something positive to focus on. My partner decided to go and inform the midwives that he felt things were developing and when would I next be checked as I was also due to go back on the monitor. I was put back on the monitor but I kept my headphones in as I didn't really want to hear what the midwife had to say. She had agreed that the surges definitely showed things were developing so my partner asked regarding the birth pool again - I was told it was not available as it was in use but she would hand over to the next midwife that I was wanting a water birth.

I am so thankful for our new midwife and also for my partner pushing for what I wanted. A new midwife came 10 minutes later and read the trace from the monitor and told me she would go and fill the pool. I had to double check I was hearing things right as I didn't want to get my hopes up if it wasn't going to happen. I was so happy, another step closer to having the birth that I had so wanted. The midwife asked to examine me and I was 4cms at 8.40pm. I can't say I was disappointed but the surges were really powerful so I would say I was surprised. I had read people who got in the pool too soon it slowed down labour so I was reluctant to get in but the midwife reassured me and suggested that I go on all 4s in the pool as she believed the baby might be back to back. I can't say I felt the relief in the pool that some people say but I think this was because things progressed pretty quickly. Surges were strong but I was getting through them and very quickly I could feel my body pushing at the end of the surge. I was a little concerned as I didn't think I could possibly be at the pushing stage, I hadn't felt the transition phase of "I can't do this" and was also doubting how I could possibly be 10cms when I had only just been examined but the midwife told me to listen to my body and if I need to push to go with it. My partner had told the midwife not to offer me pain relief unless I ask for it. I did ask at this stage for the gas and air as I wanted the mouth piece to bite down on. She asked if I wanted it switching on which I said I was happy for her to do so. I was still doing up breathing and couldn't get to grips with the gas and air so after a couple of attempts I decided to just use it to bite down on. Then my waters popped and wow did I feel that pop, I saw them shoot through the water in the pool like a jet.

During the down breathing stage I have to say I didn't feel as in control as when it was the surges. The midwives were giving advice and trying to coach me but my body totally took over and I was just going with that. She was out in 4 pushes and wow did I feel it.

We had skin to skin in the pool and delayed cord clamping, I did have the injection for the placenta delivery. My partner had skin to skin while I delivered the placenta and also was checked for tears and grazes. I didn't have anything which I was so shocked about.

We thanked our midwife later for supporting the birth that we wanted and her response was "it's your birth why shouldn't you have what you want" which was so nice and so true. We later found out that she wasn't meant to be our midwife but she had asked to have us as we wanted a water birth and she used to work in a birth center.

Adreanna and baby Aurelia

The birth of Yannis

I have to admit the last few weeks of my pregnancy had been quite a challenge. Mentally in particular, handling our patience - or better impatience. When you have your hospital bag packed, your birth preferences prepared, the nursery ready... what else is there to do but wait... and overanalyse every movement in your belly? As much as we tried to relax, we could not stop thinking about when we would finally meet our baby, well aware of the fact that first time mothers usually give birth past their due date.

It was Monday, November 15th. My due date was still one week away and I felt great - as I had throughout my pregnancy. So I went shopping with my Mum as I felt I did not have the right pyjamas for the hospital. At the same time, I decided to wash all the curtains in the living room. I did not even think this could be the nesting instinct kicking in. So I loaded the washing machine and off we went to the mall. Back home, my Mum helped me hang the curtains and I immediately loaded another machine with the pyjamas and sweat pants we had just bought just in case I would need them soon. Little had I known I would need my birth bag a few hours later.

Evening came and my husband and I had dinner and then watched the football World Championship qualifications game Bulgaria against Switzerland to distract us from our impatience. It was quite an exciting match and right before the end of the game (Bulgaria was losing 0-4), I felt a gush of warm water dripping out of me. My waters had broken. Both my husband and I remained very calm, actually both very excited with two big smiles in our faces. My only worry at that point was to leave a stain on the couch (which I didn't). So we phoned the hospital and they told us to make our way up. We arrived at the hospital by 11:30pm.

Since I had tested positive for Group B Strep a few weeks before, I knew I'd get antibiotics immediately on arrival at the hospital to prevent an infection for the baby. What I had not known, though, was the fact that a positive strep B test combined with the waters breaking according to hospital guidelines meant that I needed to be induced as no more than 24hrs should pass until the birth. So as well prepared as we felt we were, that fact had somehow not been on our radar and when the midwife, Anne, informed us about the necessary induction, we weren't utterly thrilled. That was our first aha-moment when we realized what everyone meant when they said you can be as prepared as you like for birth, it will turn out differently than you had planned. However, we did not feel as if this would happen to us and we had no other choice. We knew this was best for both baby and me and so we agreed to the procedure. I then remembered one of Claire's podcast episodes (I believe it was #27) where the guest said she and her husband told themselves 'It's coming anyway, you can't avoid it, let's do what we can'. This had somewhat become our mantra too and we smiled and kept telling ourselves 'some way or the other, that baby will come out so let's do what is best for both of us".

So I was given a propess tampon to stimulate the cervix and in addition, an IV with 250ml of penicillin every 4hrs (because of the strep B). The midwife told us to try to get some sleep and to relax for the tampon to do its magic. While my husband lay down on the couch I tried to get some sleep in bed, but I couldn't sleep at all. As I was losing so much water, the tampon kept falling out and by 4am they had to put in a new one. By 6am, the midwife realized the tampon wasn't working as I was still at 1cm. At shift change around 7am, the new midwife, Claudia, informed us that she would like to consult with my gynecologist to discuss how to proceed. She then came back and suggested we switch to the synthetic oxytocin via IV to make better progress. After using the BRAINS method and discussing with my husband, we agreed to the procedure as yet again we wanted to do what's best for the baby and me. So we had a nice breakfast to get some energy and then went to the roof top terrace of the hospital to get some final fresh air with a beautiful view over Lucerne and the lake and mountains. Around 9am, they put me on the oxytocin starting at 15ml per hour and then continuously increasing the doses in 15ml steps. I must have been at 2cm by then, however, I had written in my birth preferences that I did not want to know how much dilated I was and I really appreciated the midwife very much respecting that. The morning went on with me having minor surges that felt more like mild period cramps. By noon, I felt like I needed to breathe through the surges and I used the breathing upwards techniques we learned during our hypnobirthing course. After lunch, the midwife suggested I go into the birth pool to relax a bit. I happily agreed as I had a water birth on top of my birth preferences. In the pool, I felt amazing, weightless and able to relax. And for a moment, I was able to blend out the noisy construction works taking place right in front of the hospital. My husband was such a great support as he remained so calm, stroked my arm and back and counted backwards through the surges with me. And he kept encouraging me with how well I was doing which really motivated me and made me feel secure.

At around 2pm, the midwife suggested I come out of the tub to move around a little and try some additional positions. As I toweled myself off, I soon realized the surges were intensifying and standing on my feet felt very uncomfortable. But so did sitting, being on all fours, lying down on my side or on my back. The only position I could barely live with was sitting on the birth ball with my upper body leaning towards the bed. When that no longer seemed to work either, I moved onto the bed to lie on my side. By that time, it must have been around 3pm, my surges were getting so intense that I did not even have 30 seconds to breathe in between. I remember the bed having a handle on the side which I grabbed strongly every time a surge came and tried to breathe through it as best as I could. However, I got to a point where I could hardly bear the surges anymore. I can still hear the midwife and my husband talk to me, trying to encourage me and asking me questions, but I remember somewhat feeling like Matthew McConaughey in Interstellar, trapped behind that book case trying to speak to his daughter. I was in a complete delirium and I just could not articulate myself anymore. The oxytocin was at 75ml by then and what the midwife told us later on, it seemed I has having second stage surges and the baby was about to be born. However, apparently nothing happened down there and it was then and there when the midwife and my husband decided to stop the oxytocin from the IV for a while to give me some time to recover and breathe. I was so lucky for my husband to be there to support me and make important decisions for me in that very intense moment as I was not able to speak or think anymore due to the heavy surges. I think we did well in discussing my birth preferences so thoroughly beforehand over and over again and also agreeing on a safety word (which luckily we didn't end up needing).

It got to 4pm, it was time for another change of shifts and midwife number 3, Aleksandra arrived. She then examined me and informed us she would like to consult with my gynecologist again and would then come back to discuss our options with us. When she came back, I felt she had a sad look in her eyes and since she too knew I did not want to have any information about how dilated I was, she gently asked me if I wanted to know the current state nevertheless. I told her I assumed she was about to tell me that I had major contractions but that I still was at 2cm, and she nodded. I was exhausted and I could not understand why my body was not opening up. Yet, we remained calm and reminded ourselves of the affirmations, two of our favorite ones were "baby knows best" and "our baby will be born when our baby is ready", which helped us a lot in that moment. So with the midwife, we discussed our options. One was to go for Buscopan, an antispasmodic drug to help with the surges/cramps, but unclear whether the cervix would then open up. The other option was an epidural which would allow me to relax and breathe while at the same time my body would move forward without me physically going through all the struggle. Despite the fact that the epidural was on my "I wish not to" list on my birth preferences, we realized this was the best option we had and I was in so much need for some recharging. So by around 5pm the anesthesiologist arrived, an angel in blue I remember calling him, to place the epidural. Once it started working I felt wonderful, relieved, somehow like in a bubble... or after some glasses of bubbly.

At around 6pm, my gynecologist arrived at the hospital and very openly and kindly informed us how things would proceed. If all went well I would most probably have a natural birth within the next 6-10 hours she said. However, she also wanted us to be prepared that if my cervix would still not open, we would have to consider a caesarean by 4am the next day the very latest. We calmly took note of the information and hoped for my body to benefit from the epidural. And then, it all developed fairly quickly. I believe within 2 hours we were already at 4cm and another 1 hour later at 8cm and I didn't feel a thing. By around 10pm I was fully dilated. Our midwife told us that her shift would end soon but that she would stay until our baby is born. What an amazing human being, working extra hours because we made such a great team as she said.

The epidural was then nearly turned off so that I would feel the surges again and could help pushing. Due to the epidural, my legs got quite weak so I stayed on the bed and moved from side to side to help the baby make its way down the birth canal. I soon started to feel not only the surges, but the very strong need to push. What a magical sensation. I think this was also when the adrenaline kicked in and we realized we were soon to meet our little baby. To have enough strength to help the baby move further down I was advised to move onto my back. My gynecologist did not leave our side, I had her holding my left leg, the midwife holding my right one. And midwife number 4, Antje, who had just started her shift, assisting the birth and all three of them cheering me on. And let's not forget my amazing husband, Guido, my rock, my guardian angel, my greatest supporter who was by my side all the time, holding my hand, supporting my neck, rubbing my arm, handing me water in between the surges, cooling my forehead and neck with a cold washcloth, breathing with me, encouraging and empowering me over and over and over again. In the end, it really felt like that marathon Claire often referred to during our course and in her podcast. I felt I was surrounded by the greatest team ever, selflessly and unconditionally helping me run the race and approach the finish line

The urge to push got ever stronger and our little baby moved further and further down. I could feel its hairy little head with my fingers. My husband said he could even see the baby's head turn inside the birth canal and was absolutely fascinated by the miracle happening. A few more pushes and the baby's head was born. The midwife encouraged me to instantly push one or two more times and the body was born too. November 16th, 11:30pm. I believe they call it the ejection reflex as little baby was literally catapulted away from me. As I heard our baby's voice for the first time I was in tears, in complete awe of the miracle of mother nature, so, so happy, speechless. We had not known the gender until then and I heard my husband say to me in tears "It's Yannis, it's Yannis, it's Yannis! " What a wonderful moment, I can't even describe in words how we felt. Our little boy had the cord around his neck, the midwife said. Once the cord had stopped pulsating my husband cut it and then they put Yannis on my chest and I could hold him for the first time. I still get tears while typing this. The most magical sensation I have ever felt. I was no longer a women, I was a mother now. We had so much time for bonding while somewhere in another world the placenta was born. Baby boy even managed to latch for the first time while on my chest. I remember holding his back with my left hand and it felt we were almost glued together with the sticky vernix still all over his body. I would never ever let him go anymore, that was clear.

Our birth has been the most wonderful experience for all three of us. Hypnobirthing helped us so much in getting all the knowledge around what physically happens during birth. That knowledge really empowered us during birth to make informed decisions and to stay calm and positive at all times. Looking back at my birth preferences, almost everything I had noted on the "I wish not to" list had in the end happened (being induced, having a permanent CTG, an epidural, giving birth on my back etc.). However, we always felt empowered and calm. Not for one single moment did we feel forced to take any decision nor pushed towards a certain solution and the whole birth, despite taking almost 26 hours, never turned hectic. I truly believe that Yannis could feel the calm environment he was born into. He is such a calm, happy baby. He sleeps a lot and literally never cries or screams and we feel so blessed.

Thank you Claire for all your wonderful help and support, also during the time our baby had not yet turned head down and we thought our baby was breech. I am convinced the meditations and visualizations helped our baby turn in time and made us remain positive. Your podcast as well as our 4-week course have been instrumental in helping us have an amazing birth experience. We cannot thank you enough, dear Claire.

Seraina and baby Yannis

WATER BIRTH

The birth of Frieda

We found out that I was pregnant with our second daughter in December, just after our first daughter's 4th birthday. Although we always wanted a second child I had mixed feelings. My first birth was a very traumatic experience, and although I had a lot of counselling already to process it and manage the post-traumatic stress it still wasn't easy. A birth trauma is quite a special kind of trauma, as despite the experience a lot of us decide to do it again anyway! You wouldn't get into another car crash on purpose!

I worked hard and was very lucky to be able to organise myself a very good support network throughout my pregnancy. I got referred to the perinatal mental health team and they put me in touch with a brilliant counsellor who supported me until after the birth. I also decided to contact a private midwife to take over my antenatal care. This is pretty expensive, but it was so extremely helpful to gain some sense of trust and security again, as each appointment was face to face at my home, lasting up to one hour. Once I got to know and trust her, I decided that I also wanted to have this midwife attending the birth. I didn't feel confident enough to go for a home birth, which she could have done, but she managed to convince the head midwife at our hospital to attend in a doula role despite the fact that Covid restrictions would normally only allow one birth partner at that time.

While processing my trauma, I already had it in my mind that I would look into hypnobirthing more if I ever got pregnant again. I bought an online course and got through most of it. During my daily walks I listened to The Hypnobirthing Podcast and also a positive birth stories podcast. I learned so much about physiological birth and better understood what set me up for the experience I had the first time around. The women who talked about the pride and strength they got out of their births started to shift my mind set to imagine the upcoming birth as a positive and powerful experience. For coping strategies, I drew a lot of inspirations from the fact that I used to do rock climbing and have also run two half marathons. Each of these are experiences where I pushed my body to go further, even though part of me would think about giving up. It reminded me that I really wouldn't feel the pain so much while trying to grab the next hold or doing the sprint for the finishing line. That all showed me that I indeed have the ability to change my mind-set around the pain during labour and therefore not experience it as this overwhelming negative thing. In addition, I did regular yoga sessions thinking a lot about the positions I would like to use during labour as well as the breathing techniques. It really helped calm my nerves in the weeks leading up to the big day and in getting things ready for the big day: writing my birth plan, creating a birth playlist with comforting and happy songs, printing out affirmations and colouring them in together with my daughter, choosing my birthing outfit, buying the snacks to keep me going during labour.

My husband tried his best to support me through this second pregnancy, but it wasn't always easy for him to understand the trauma and how I was dealing with it. It was hard for him to understand why I wouldn't just go for the elective caesarean. He listened to some of the hypnobirthing classes with me and my suggestions of what he could do during labour. In general, as with my first, the pregnancy was healthy. There was a stressful period, when baby decided to settle into a breech position for a very long period. My midwife was not a fan of vaginal breech birth and was nudging me to think about the elective caesarean. At that point I was VERY set on vaginal birth without interventions and tried everything to get baby to flip, long walks, inversions, bouncing on the birth ball daily. By 36 weeks, magically and without me even noticing, she had turned head down.

In the evening before my due date I felt some very mild cramps very low in my abdomen. I got quite excited, joking to my husband that baby might be a typical punctual German (as I am), born on her due date. But the next morning the cramping is gone. I was disappointed but remind myself that my midwife had mentioned that second babies quite commonly move in and out of the pelvis several times before birth and this can trigger cramping.

In the days to follow I ate lots of dates, drank raspberry leaf tea, ate hot curry, went on plenty of walks and did random "labour inducing" workouts on YouTube. I have another crampy night three days later, but still not the real thing. I am starting to get slightly panicky, because I am past my due date by now and per guidelines my midwife has to start talking about inductions. She offers me a membrane sweep at our next appointment, but in the end I decide not to do it, as I am feeling that things are happening already and also with the understanding that there are some risks to this procedure.

At 40+5, again cramping starts in the evening. While bouncing on the birth ball, I debate with myself whether I should stay up or go for a walk, in case that could help to move things along. But I decide to go to bed anyway, thinking that if nothing is starting this night, I will just be very tired. I manage to sleep, but I wake up a couple of times from cramping. At 5am the next morning, the cramps are still there, and I just know that I am properly in the latent phase now. I get up, quite excited, and start to bake muffins. I text the babysitter to let her know that she'll probably will have to take our daughter tonight. I make breakfast for everyone, we eat and my husband takes our daughter to nursery. The contractions are mild down in my abdomen, but regular. I text my midwife just before 10am, letting her know that things have started. I also start losing some mucus in bits, also quite a bit of blood. I can't decide whether this is fresh blood or not, but decide not to tell anyone, as it doesn't look worrying to me and I don't want to alarm anyone. I also phone the midwife-led unit, the place where I am planning to give birth, to let them know that I am in early labour.

I put on my favourite movie, bounce on the birth ball and start to time contractions a bit. They are 4-5 minutes apart lasting 30-40 seconds and I can talk and do things. My husband keeps himself busy around the house, but I prefer to have time on my own. At around 1pm, we have some sandwiches for lunch and go for a 20 minute walk. I can still talk and walk through contractions, but have to focus a bit more now. Once back home, I put on another movie, but 30 minutes in, I realise that I can't focus on it anymore and I switch it off. I fiddle around with my phone a bit and find a nice setup where I listen to my birth playlist on the headphones, but during a contraction I use an app that times contractions and also iterates a count for breathing. I find this counting surprisingly helpful and spend the next hour like that, kneeling over the birthing ball, eyes closed. My husband wants to know whether he should do anything. I let him set up a charger for the phone and get me drinks, but then send him away, as I prefer to be on my own focusing on breathing and keep the contractions going. They are now after the walk definitely ramping up, every 3-4 minutes lasting 40-50 seconds.

At 3pm, I call my midwife, as the app tells me I might be in established labour and I know she needs more than 1 hour to make her way to ours. When she arrives she checks my blood pressure and baby. My contractions all of a sudden are all over the place, spacing out to 8 minutes apart or not lasting long at all. I panic, thinking I need to "show some proper labour", now that I called her out. But then I remind myself to calm down, that such thinking is stressful and unhelpful. I pop on my headphones again and return to my labour bubble. Within 10 minutes or so my contractions are back on track. I find this very re-assuring that I can help my contractions by staying calm and focused and that the things I heard in the hypnobirthing class do work. They intensify now, every 3-4 minutes lasting 1 minute and I start to become a bit vocal, moaning. Just after 5pm, the midwife suggests to leave for the hospital as she has the impression things move quite quickly. I call the midwife-led unit, but unfortunately, they tell me that there is no room for me ready yet and ask whether I want to wait. But as we are certain that we have to leave now or have the baby at home, we refuse and are told to go to delivery suite for now.

We are only a 15min drive away from the hospital, I have several contractions in the car. My husband drops me in front of the entrance, then drives off to park the car. I am stepping a bit to the side behind a construction fence, as I feel quite conscious about having contractions in plain daylight with people going in and out of the hospital. My husband and my midwife come with the luggage and we find our way upstairs. I keep having contractions, moaning more, I have to lean on someone or walls for support. In the delivery suite we are shown to a small room with a bed. My husband immediately reminds me to not lie on it and helps me to get the backrest up. I kneel over it facing the wall. It all starts to feel a bit overwhelming, so I pop my headphones back on and manage to mostly filter out what is happening behind me. Contractions are every 2-3 minutes, lasting about 1 minute and are still getting more intense. I grab onto a rail at the back of the bed, and start to get really loud now, roaring. It surprises me how much the roaring really helps to get through the contractions. At some point, my husband starts to massage my lower back and I really love that. After 30 minutes or so we still haven't been seen by anyone from the hospital, so my midwife (who is now just in her doula role and has no clinical responsibility) decides to get someone, as she feels things are moving quickly. The responsible midwife comes in and tells me that I have to have a vaginal check to be allowed to stay on delivery suite. I am pretty irritated by the wording but don't get a chance to even think about an answer, as the next contraction comes. So I just hold up my hand, not even meaning that as an aggressive gesture, but just to signal that I can't talk because of the contraction. She doesn't address me again and I later learn from my midwife, that after observing me for a few minutes, she agreed that I was clearly in active labour and didn't need to be checked. There is also someone trying for several minutes to take my temperature with a metal stick under my arm and fails, which I find pretty annoying. In general, all is very busy and distracting, but my contractions keep coming nevertheless, very powerful and intense. I keep grabbing the bed rails and roar. I feel safe and grateful, that I can fully rely on my husband and midwife to sort out whatever is going on behind my back. They do the talking and protect me from too much intrusion, so I can keep focusing on labouring. This feels so valuable and good and is crucial for me not to panic in this not ideal situation. My midwife also repeats a few affirmations, my husband keeps reminding me to relax in between contractions. Just hearing those familiar voices throughout is very calming. He also keeps offering me food and drink, I only manage sips of coconut water and smoothies at this point.

Then, finally, we get the OK to go to the midwife-led unit. I walk over leaning on walls and probably screaming through contractions in the corridor, but this is bit of a blur. We arrive in a small room, dimly lit with purple light, a bed, a small pool, it is really nice and cosy. Someone says "what about some pethidine" as soon as we enter the room, and I am a bit annoyed by as my birth plan clearly states "don't offer me pain relief, I will ask for it, when I need it". My midwife immediately jumps in though and deals with them. I get on the bed and lean over the birth ball once again, while they start to fill the pool. I think it is at this point that I have the transition, because I remember thinking or even saying, that this is so hard, I am not sure how much longer I can do this. But that moment passes very quickly.

The pool is ready and I get in and it feels very relaxing and nice. I am back on my knees and contractions are super strong now, but I don't remember ever feeling a big urge to push. I am still roaring, holding onto some handles on the side of the pool. The local midwife tells me to stop screaming but rather use that energy to push down, which I find very hard to do initially, as my instinct tells me not to go there. After a while my midwife asks me to turn around into a squat. This new position feels really uncomfortable and I say "I hate that". Later she explains to me, that she felt a more upright position would help move baby, as the intense contractions were going on for a while already and she was worried that I wouldn't be able to last much longer. I also think it is at this point that the local midwife asks all of a sudden whether baby is head down, as they actually hadn't checked. My midwife assures them that she felt baby head down and we had a scan at 37 weeks confirming that. They ask me to check myself. I reach down and feel first the squashy membranes as my waters still haven't gone at that point and poking further with my finger I feel something hard, which I assume is the head and I say so.

Still, contractions are coming strong and now that I actively push under the guidance of the local midwife, not screaming but keeping it in, I can feel baby crowning. What I can't see, but my husband tells me later is that they can see the membranes bulging out like a balloon and going in again, as head moves towards the exit and back again. I hear my husband saying "this is so cool" with a big smile on his face and this is very reassuring and positive for me. This part feels physically very challenging, as I can feel the head crowning (the famous 'ring of fire') but not quite going through yet and once the contraction is over, it goes back. In my head I know I have to try really hard so I put all my energy in it and everyone is shouting to keep going and then all of a sudden I feel the head pop out. That is the best feeling ever, as I know that was the hard part. I am told later, that my waters broke just before the head is born. I am relaxing and with the next contraction baby's body just wiggles out in this corkscrew movement I've seen in some of the birthing videos. I reach for her in the water and lift her out myself (something I really wanted to do, even had it in my birth plan). Someone says the cord is around the neck and I very calmly unwind it myself (probably with the help of the midwives) and lift her up to my chest. I am absolutely overjoyed that she is here with me and just came out like that without any complications. Overall I was in the pool just about 25 minutes, before she was born at 7.14pm.

While I am enjoying this moment with my little girl, my midwife is commenting that she is a bit worried about the blood in the pool water. The local midwife is not, but they suggest the injection for the placenta anyway. My plan was to have a natural third stage, but at this point I am in the "I don't care" mood and say yes. Someone takes baby, my husband clamps the cord, and they ask me to sit up on the edge of the pool. I am very exhausted and need some help with that. I get the injection and then they ask me to do some coughing to help them get the placenta out. All is good and I get out of the pool onto the bed. We have our first feed and enjoy the 'Golden hour' undisturbed. Later I need some stitching and my husband and the little one wait in another room for me. Back with them, I enjoy how well I feel compared to after my first birth, as I am able to walk around and have a shower right away.

Overall, I definitely got the positive birth experience I was working so hard for. It was very intense, physically exhausting, but the thought afterwards was "It was just the right amount I could cope with. I am happy that it was so intense and quick because I could handle it but wouldn't have wanted to handle it much longer". Also I barely thought about pain relief, basically only before I entered the pool during transition. Of course, there was luck in it as well, as I had no complications. The biggest difference compared to my first birth was for sure my mind-set. I am certain the intensity of the contractions wasn't any different to my first birth and they definitely felt the most powerful whole-body experience imaginable for me. But while I can definitely remember how they physically felt from my first birth and specifically the pain, I actually can't remember the ones from the second time around. My brain has just processed those completely differently as something non-threatening and therefore no need to keep it. And I can't emphasise enough how important it was to have my midwife there as an advocate, who could shield me completely from all the room availability discussions, potential interventions and so on. I could just focus on my labour and managed to let go of all anxiety and fears, and I am convinced that this resulted in this rather quick labour. I would totally do it again and this time I would plan it as a home birth. If it wouldn't be for pregnancy, which I definitely don't want to do again.

Sandra and baby Frieda

The birth of Willow

On Saturday 9th November Chris, Nicky (Chris' mother) and I went to the Polo club in the evening. Just before we left I had started wearing a liner as I felt there was some water coming out. While we were at the Polo Club I started to get stronger Braxton Hicks contractions than I had felt previously. So much so that I warned Chris and also messaged Sophie, one of our midwives. We didn't stay out too long and headed home to wait and see if anything happened. Nothing happened. Chris and I went to bed early, we were both exhausted, and ended up having a big 9hr sleep.

Sunday morning I woke up and instead of having my breakfast first, which I ALWAYS do, I decided I needed to walk. I walked a couple of kilometres around the plot – I tracked the walk and noticed that I was walking 2minutes per km slower than usual. I felt so heavy and the baby felt so low in my pelvis. The previous days I was walking 4-6km daily to try and get things moving but today I could only manage 2km.

At 1:30pm I was sitting on the sofa while Chris was making lasagne. I stood up to get something and my waters broke with a huge gush – just like in the movies. I hadn't been having any contractions so I was quite surprised. I wasn't sure what to do so I stood there saying "oh my god" while Chris laughed and then led me to the bathroom. I stood in the shower while more water came out and Chris let the midwives know.

The midwives suggested I eat and rest before things get going. Chris looked up that it can take up to 48hrs for labour to proceed after waters break! I lay in bed but I was way too excited to nap. I listened to the Hollie De Cruz daily relaxation and tried to keep my breathing steady. I messaged Jo (my stepmother) and asked her to come over and bring the cake she and Jamie (my sister) had baked.

Jo arrived and at a similar time some contractions had started, they were just like the Braxton Hicks but with a little more of the cramping sensation. By 5pm when a surge came I had to close my eyes and ride it out – it was a little more intense but I could still carry on a conversation in between. We were sitting on the veranda in the afternoon light and I had the dogs either side of me. The surges were coming around 10 minutes apart. Nicky left with Jo at around 6pm and Chris ran me a bath. The mothers said that I should probably head to the hospital soon but I really didn't believe them! I was so worried about being sent home again; turns out they were right though.

I put on my Yoga Relaxation playlist and got in our bath tub, the water felt amazing! We were using an app to record the surges which made everything so easy. While I was in the water Chris packed the car, had a shower, tidied the house and kept checking in on me. I remember telling him that I wasn't in any pain but that each surge was an intensity I couldn't liken to anything else. The surges are just like waves, you can feel them coming and they build up before slowing down. It's a powerful feeling.

Chris was outside repositioning the car closer to the house and I got out of the bath and went into the bedroom. A surge came and I lay on the bed in child's pose. I felt a huge relief in my lower back. Both Ndito and Morani (our dogs) stayed by my side for the entire duration of early labour. They knew something was happening. When Chris came back inside I said to him that I think we need to leave for the hospital now. Surges were coming every 3-5minutes at this stage and the app told us we were in established labour. It was 7:45pm when we left home.

The car journey to the hospital was almost unbearable towards the end. I don't mean to sound dramatic but it was very difficult for me to stay focused and the surges were coming faster and harder each time. I hated being confined to the seat and it felt stuffy. Poor Chris, he was driving the car in rush hour traffic and I was squeezing his arm through each surge and trying to keep my eyes closed so as not to be frustrated with the traffic. Every light was red. The road was so busy. We were just getting to Arusha when I said to Chris that I needed to get out of the car NOW. I just felt like it was time and things were happening. And I could not be in the car anymore. Chris didn't let me out but kept reassuring me that we would be there soon.

We arrived at the hospital a little after 8:30pm. I got out of the car but soon found that I couldn't walk, the surges were coming too fast. Sophie and Chris brought me a wheelchair and I sat in it and covered my face with my scarf while they wheeled me all the way up to the birthing room. The hospital was bright and loud and busy so I was very grateful to be able to cover my face and pretend I was still at home! The midwives had everything ready for me in the room, they were the best. The pool was inflated and filled perfectly. Mahela helped me undress down to my bikini top, Sophie quickly and gently did a vaginal examination (I didn't want to be told how dilated I was so the midwives kept it between them) and I stepped into the pool. Later I was told that I was 5cm dilated when we arrived and I progressed to 10cm in 1 hour.

Again, the water felt amazing! It just supported my whole body and took away so much of the tension. I asked Chris to turn off the lights and just like that I was back in my zone. It felt like there was no time at all between the surges.

I had no time to put up my positive affirmation posters that my girlfriends and I had made. The pool was even more comfortable than the bath because the inflatable floor and sides meant I could move into different positions very easily. The intensity increased immediately and I began to shout, roar and scream my way up and down each wave. I had imagined that I would be silent in labour due to my yoga, meditation and hypnobirthing practice like some serene goddess, but I was loud on another level! It helped me to keep focused and also keep my face and jaw relaxed. I told Chris "it's here" at the beginning of each surge and then surrendered to the feeling of it. I felt my body relaxing and opening.

There was a brief period where I got out of the pool because I felt hot. It didn't last long as I needed the relief and support of the water to help me during the surges. I couldn't be in the position I wanted out of the water. In the pool I mainly was on my hands and knees, or squatting and using the side of the pool to lean on. The pool had a little inflatable seat on it which the midwives asked me to sit on a couple of times so they could see better. Sophie helped me with some massage a few times between surges. It felt amazing. I had my eyes closed almost the entire time. I did not take my hand off Chris. I needed him to anchor me, to be there beside me the whole time. Between surges Chris gave me cool water to drink, every single chance he got he gave me water. We had talked about how important it would be for me to stay hydrated. He was amazing. He didn't talk (apparently I told him he wasn't allowed) but he was there for me and when I was losing track of my breath he grounded me by breathing like we had practiced. He was my safety, he was my protector and the only connection I wanted to the world. I didn't need to worry about anything else because he was there and he knew what I wanted and I trusted him absolutely.

He later told me that when the surge came I was trying to bite his fingers (oops!) and almost ripped his clothes, I don't remember these things! I remember kissing his hands and stroking his arm between waves, I remember I felt so connected to him, I remember thanking him over and over. I remember he was there, fully there, with me the entire time. I think during the intensity of the wave I was so focused inwards, I was completely surrendering to the process I wasn't aware of anything in the room. It was so animalistic, so primal. I felt so powerful and so in control somehow. Even though I wasn't in control of the surges.

Throughout labour I spoke to myself and my baby out loud. I told myself it was ok, I was strong, I said I wasn't afraid. I kept saying "It's ok my baby, we're together and I love you". I remember reading in the days leading up to labour not to forget that your baby is also going through it with you, remember to connect and reassure your baby. I could feel Willow getting lower in my body and each time her heart rate was checked she was steady, I believe she was calm.

I had no concept of time. It could have been minutes or hours. I don't know. But Mahela asked me if I felt like I needed to poo. I did. The midwives told me it's time to start pushing – our baby was ready to start coming down the birth canal.

It felt amazing to start pushing. I pushed for a while. I kept asking if they could see her head and they couldn't, Sophie said she would tell me when she could. Finally she said "Hannah look on the next contraction and you will see your baby's head". I did. I saw her head. Oh my god. My baby! I gently touched the top of her head with my finger and kept saying "my baby my baby". Chris was worried I would hurt her but I was touching so gently, she was almost here. I was feeling a little bit tired but seeing her head gave me new energy. I pushed and pushed and pushed and she got a little bit closer each time. I could feel her head coming in and out during each surge. There was a strong stinging feeling but mostly it felt so right.

Sophie told me to use the full contraction and to listen to my body. I used my breath to direct my pushing to where I could feel her head. But then her head got stuck half in and half out. This was very, very uncomfortable. The midwives wanted me to lay on my back in the water but I wanted to be on my hands and knees so we were clashing a little.

Sophie decided it was time to help because she had been stuck for a little while, "you're going to have to get out of the pool so we can see what's going on". Chris helped me stand up. All the while Mahela was checking Willow's heartrate and Willow stayed calm and steady. She didn't get distressed at all. I spoke to her the whole time – I told her it's ok my baby, we are nearly there. It's ok, it's ok, it's ok.

When I was standing it was really uncomfortable, my perineum was stretched and I was trying not to push in between the waves. I heard Sophie say to Mahela "we're going to have to do an episiotomy". I really didn't want an episiotomy. I really believed that Willow was about to come and I trusted my feeling. I just needed to wait for the next surge. I said "No, no, no! Don't cut me! Don't cut me, I can do it. I can do it! Let me do it!" and I tried to escape from them. Sophie was behind me so I couldn't see what she was doing and that made me a little nervous. I knew that she didn't need to cut me, I could feel that Willow was coming, I just knew it somehow. On the next surge Willow's head came out. I reached down and felt her little cheeks. She was facing my inner thigh instead of backwards which is why I had felt so much pressure in my back.

I pushed one more time and Sophie helped me catch her and pulled her up on my chest. She was so slimy! She was completely covered in vernix. She cried immediately! But the second I held her she stopped and she was so alert, she was looking at me and clasping her hand around my bikini strap.

The time was 12am on the 11th, her due date, just as her dad had predicted all along (I will never hear the end of this!).

Now the midwives wanted to check how I had torn, they were sure it would be a bad tear as they had wanted the episiotomy. I agreed to the syntocinon injection to help me birth the placenta more quickly. The placenta came out whole, and once the cord had stopped pulsing Chris cut it. He was adamant he wouldn't cut it but when the moment came he changed his mind! I was holding Willow the whole time and Chris had put on her playlist that I had made so I could sing to her. In this moment I felt I could never ever let her go. She was part of my heart, I can't describe the love I felt in any other way.

Mahela used a gauze to stop the bleeding and when she could see she said it wasn't bad at all, she would just need to do two stitches. When she was done, she cleaned me and I got to hold Willow for an hour and a half before Mahela gave her to Chris and then I went through to have a shower. There was no hot water so I just had to have a little bucket shower using water from the kettle. There was still a lot of blood coming out of me which was normal. My belly was like a partially deflated balloon. And it stung a lot when I peed but apart from that I felt high!

Willow was so content with Chris. He was holding her on his bare chest and she was still looking around so curious. The midwives cleaned up the bathroom and emptied the pool and then left us to it. We were now three. We had the music playing and the fairy lights on and just lay there – Willow and me on the hospital bed and Chris on a mattress on the floor. I could barely sleep but I lay there with Willow on my belly kissing and kissing her little hands and little face.

Hannah and baby Willow

The birth of Xander

This was my second birth using hypnobirthing and I have to credit Claire at The Nurture Nest for providing me with all the tools for a positive labour and birth experience.

We had planned a home birth this time, my first had been a hospital birth, however at 37 weeks my local authority suspended home births due to a lack of staff. I was initially really disappointed but this was completely out of our control and so we decided on our local birth centre instead.

The morning of Saturday 14th August 2021 I was a day over my due date and I thought it was still going to be several days until the baby arrived. I had lost my mucus plug a few weeks before but since then I had only felt a few tightenings here and there. My partner (Dom), 2 year old daughter and I spent the morning taking a long walk around the lake close to where we live and the afternoon relaxing at home.

Just after 10pm I had turned out the light to go to sleep when I heard a 'pop' noise. I gasped and made Dom jump and told him I thought my waters had just broken. I went to the bathroom to check the colour of the waters. During my first birth my daughter had meconium in her waters and I knew if this were to happen again I wouldn't be able to give birth at the local birthing centre. Thankfully they looked clear! We called the birthing centre to advise my waters had broken and they invited us to come in to check. I called my Dad to come and collect my daughter, got dressed and packed the last few bits in our bags. I remember saying to my Dad to take his time and not to rush as it would probably be a while as at this point my contractions had not started.

I arrived at Maidstone Birth Centre at around 11pm and was assessed. They did some quick observations of me and baby but did not examine me at this point. My contractions had now started and were manageable using hypnobirthing techniques. We were invited to stay at the birth centre to see how things progressed but at this point I assumed it could still be a while yet and decided it would be better to go home and get some rest.

We arrived back home about 11:45pm and my contractions had started to ramp up and so I got Dom to attach the TENS machine. I tried to lie down on the bed but could not get comfortable and the only place I seemed to be able to get comfy was in the bathroom sat on the toilet in the dark or pacing on the landing. I felt that something had changed in the short time we had been home and my contractions were coming closing together and building in intensity. I knew I wanted to go back to the birth centre and so Dom called to let them know that we would be heading back in. So at 00:30 we got back into the car. There is a great video of me on our Ring doorbell coming back out of the house and heading to the car. I had to dig deep on the car journey back, although it's not even 10 minutes away I was not comfortable being sat in the car and worked hard to maintain my calm breathing and visualisation to get through the journey.

When we arrived back at the birth centre I remember feeling relieved that I could hear the water running to fill up the birth pool and straight away asking if I could go to the toilet (my happy place) I sat down on the toilet and the midwife took one look at me and said 'I think we need to get you off the toilet as baby is coming'. The midwife helped me undress and I stood for a few contractions standing and leaning against the window sill. The midwife then said if I wanted to get into the pool I needed to go quickly as baby would be with us really soon. I got into the pool at round 00:50 and sat on my knees leaning against the side using the gas and air to breathe through the contractions. At this point my partner had set-up his phone to play our hypnobirthing music and to video the birth. During the birth of our daughter he had taken loads of photographs which was so great for me to look at afterwards so I wanted to make sure we had that again and it was even better having the video this time too.

I laboured in the pool for just under 20 minutes. I had two midwives with me the whole time, encouraging me to do little pushes, keep my shoulders down and relaxed and body in the water. I shut my eyes and tried to focus on breathing baby down with each contraction. After a short time pushing, Xander was born in the water at 01:08 Sunday 15th August weighing 9lb 12oz. Xander poo'd the moment he was born and so we had to get out of the water for our first cuddle and because of this he needed to be monitored for the first 12 hours just to ensure he hadn't swallowed any meconium.

I felt exhausted and sore after the birth. It had all happened so quickly I needed a moment just to process what had happened. It had been just 3 hours from my waters breaking to my son being born and I felt a little in shock. After some tea and toast I felt better and ready for a cuddle. We moved from the birthing room into a private room where the 3 of us stayed overnight. After a few more checks the 3 of us headed home to introduce Xander to his big sister.

Debbie and baby Xander

The birth of Charlie

When I read about hypnobirthing early in my pregnancy and having done a fair bit of meditation in previous years, it instantly appealed to my appreciation of the power of the mind and the power of breathing. It also appealed to my fascination with the human body and what it's capable of. I went on to do a hypnobirthing course at 28 weeks and then practiced techniques every other day. I also listened to The Nurture Nest hypnobirthing podcast which was invaluable as well.

It all started as I had literally put my phone down on the bedside table after texting some friends just before 11.30pm. I remember being laid on my side and feeling only a couple of mild period cramps roughly 10 minutes apart and wondering if this was it. I was 41 +1 so I knew it could be anytime. I had read that if it feels like period cramps, then try rolling over or moving around as they might get stronger if it's the real deal. Well this worked! As I rolled onto my back, they instantly changed from that period cramp sensation to what I knew were real contractions. When you know, you certainly do know!

I felt a little nervous but the overriding feeling was excitement not only for the baby's arrival but also for the challenge of labour. I felt powerful and had such a strong sense of determination to come out the other side with a positive labour to look back on and smile about.

I quietly woke my husband Harry, to let him know that labour had started but then told him to go back to sleep as he was going to need it! I went through to the spare bedroom, knelt down on all fours which felt the most comfortable and started breathing (in through my nose for 4 and out through my mouth for 8) alongside my visualisations I'd practiced. I found a sunrise image worked well for me in order to keep me focused and feel calmer. I phoned triage to let them know my labour had started and then spent the next 90 minutes or so practicing my breathing but also running back and forth to the toilet! I'd read that your body can often expel everything it doesn't need during early labour and this was very true for me! I will never forget holding onto the wall with one hand and the sink with the other, bracing myself for the next contraction!

I woke Harry around 1am and then I distinctly remember being leant over the end of our bed when I phoned my Mum to come and collect our dog, Stanley. Harry packed the final bits for our hospital bags, gathered up everything the dog would need for the next few days at my Mums and then packed our car. I opened the Freya app to start recording my contractions as I had the sudden realisation they were coming thick and fast without much rest in between. I had to do a double check, when I was already having 3 within 10 minutes for around a minute each by 1.30am. In my head it just seemed too quick for some reason. I'd always imagined I'd be at home for hours and hours playing the impatient waiting game. But the pain had also ramped up to levels I was struggling to cope with too so I then knew it was time to go to hospital.

Thinking back to the sight of me on all fours in the back of our car driving to the hospital at 2am is comical. I kept looking out of the back window to see if I was giving anyone some memorable laughs in the cars behind but luckily the roads were pretty empty as it was a normal early Wednesday morning in March.

We arrived and I quickly reverse crawled out of the car (accidentally hitting the car next to us with the door oops).

Harry somehow thought it was better to run to the boot to unload the car than to help his labouring wife out of the backseat which will forever make me laugh. I left Harry at the car and almost ran to the doors of the labour ward before the next contraction hit. Harry caught up with me inside when I was being held at the second set of security doors. This next bit is still a bit hazy and confusing but we think a couple of young nurses stumbled upon us and let us in through the doors into the delivery ward when we actually should have walked further along to triage. When one of the midwives then saw me gliding towards her bent over in a wheelchair, she seemed pretty flustered from what I remember as we later learnt the delivery ward was very busy. She decided not to send us to triage thankfully for some reason and put us into delivery room 1.

Debbie, my midwife, asked me up onto the bed to examine me around 2.30am and I was 3cm. After that I was keen not to be on my back again as the pain seemed a lot worse in that position for me. So I happily spent the next few hours stood up and leant over the side of the bed. During these hours, Harry put some battery tea lights on, we dimmed the lights and I tried the TENS machine and yoga ball (both seemed to make the pain worse so they were big no no's). I also can't forget the near miss of the cardboard vomit bowl over the bed. Luckily a midwife thrust it under my head just in time. Sounds crazy but I loved seeing my body seemingly expelling everything it didn't need, again, just as I had read.

During contractions I barked orders at Harry to massage and compress my lower back with all of his body force that he could muster, to help alleviate some of the intensity. My contractions were all in my back, not at the front. Strangely, during contractions I didn't seem to get much rest either as the sensations seemed to linger and ache.

At 4.30am I reluctantly crawled onto the bed to be examined again and I was now 6cm. My waters then broke while I was still up on the bed. I had managed the pain well up until now with only loud, deep breathing but that next contraction after my waters had broken forced the first scream out of me before I even realised I had made a noise haha! I later learnt that this is when the baby's head is now pushing down with more force on your cervix without the cushion of your amniotic fluid. Debbie and Harry quickly reminded me to return to my breathing and visualisations. This was a huge help and I was straight back to focusing on my deep breaths. Debbie rushed off to run the water as I'd decided on a water birth if I could. In hindsight I could have actually gotten in the pool sooner but I don't think they had expected me to dilate to 6cm so quickly. As I was going for a wee before entering the pool, I got my bloody show. Again as strange as it sounds, I remember thinking 'there's another amazing and clever thing that my body just unconsciously did as predicted it would'.

When I got in the pool around 5am, the soothing sensations and instant relief were unbelievable. I was offered gas and air and jumped at the chance. This combined with the buoyancy of the water was like a double whammy of pain relief. It felt incredible. I must have relaxed enough to finally notice the silence in the room around me and so I asked for Harry to put some calming music on.

On reflection I wish I'd have asked Harry to video some of my time in the pool. I was apparently spouting hilarious nonsense and blurting things out like how I had no idea 'how cavewomen did this without any pain relief'! I would also have loved to see the movements my body was making. I remember a very strong thrusting sensation that almost pushed me up out of the pool and over the side each time it came over me. These were accompanied by what I'd call very primal sounding deep grunts. This happened a few times before I asked the midwife if it was normal, which obviously it was but I'd never seen any woman move dramatically upwards in the way it felt I was. It wasn't until the thrusting sensations intensified that I realised I must be in the down stage of labour and must be pushing the baby through the birth canal. It's amazing that I genuinely have barely any memory of any pain during these 'thrusts' or my time in the pool. So much for the active stages of labour increasing in pain intensity - for me anyway!

45 minutes after entering the pool, Debbie said that I needed to get out as the baby's heartbeat was slowing. I remember when I had originally lowered myself into the pool, I had had the thought of 'nobody is getting me out of this pool and if they dare to try, they'll be met with fury'! However once I heard the baby was in danger, I immediately climbed out without a second thought or ask. Harry always loves telling people how I apparently looked like Mr Staypuft from the film Ghostbusters - quickly throwing myself out of the pool and nakedly stomping my way back across the delivery ward to our room, with Debbie trying to keep my modesty with a towel wrapped around me. I put my black oversized top back on and was helped onto the bed. Debbie called for other midwives and I remember overhearing a conversation about them needing to find some local anesthetic as they were going to have to perform an episiotomy to get the baby out fast. I will never forget thinking 'okay yeah sure, you go for it, this baby is going to be out before anyone makes it back with any anesthetic'. How true that was. Again it was amazing to witness and feel my body knowing exactly what was happening and how close I was to delivering.

One last big push and here he was! 5.47am. It still blows my mind how fast I must have dilated those last 4cm in the space of around an hour. I never even knew that was possible, especially for your first, but apparently so. The midwife then told me it was a boy and placed him on me. I hugged him tight and kept saying over and over how gorgeous he was. He really did look absolutely perfect! Sadly they then had to quickly cut the cord which was sooner than I'd have liked but I didn't really mind as I just wanted him to be healthy and safe. They took him through to another room with Harry following. Debbie told me they just needed to give him some oxygen as he was a little too pale. She checked me over after delivering the placenta and I had no tears or need for stitches, even with a fast delivery, which I still can't quite believe. That had been one of my biggest worries and fears and the recovery of that afterwards. Never underestimate the power of eating 3 medjool dates a day combined with perineal massage from week 34! I am convinced that is why I didn't tear.

5 minutes after Charlie had left, a different midwife came in to tell me everything was fine and asked if I had a name for him yet. Me and Harry had previously discussed a few options but had never settled on one although I just knew it was to be Charlie. Harry had said he loved it too but I basically didn't give him the chance to agree for the final go ahead. Charlie was only gone 10 minutes or so and was soon back in my arms, healthy and well.

We were and are totally obsessed. We couldn't stop staring at him and were in complete awe. All his little movements and noises were the cutest things we'd ever seen. Thanks to hypnobirthing I really did get the smooth, quick, calm and incredible labour that I had envisioned many times in the months prior. The power of envisioning your goals and future is never to be underestimated.

Kate and baby Charlie

The birth of Dylan

I did a hypnobirthing course at 22 weeks and listened to my affirmations going to bed. I also listened to The Hypnobirthing Podcast and only allowed positive birth stories into my headspace. My waters broke just before midnight on 29th December. I was awake most of the night with very manageable surges, using the Freya app to count my breaths. I got some sleep and took my dog for a walk. By midday on 30th December the surges seemed to slow down so I called the hospital just to let them know my waters had gone and to see what they advised. They told me to go into hospital to check on baby and make sure it was my definitely my waters that had gone. They confirmed all was well, sent me home and told me to come back at 6am the next day if I hadn't progressed to established labour, for an induction. At this point I was again having some manageable surges.

I went home, had some lunch, got in the bath around 3:30pm and was practicing my hypnobirthing breathing and, well I progressed very quickly after that. I got out of the bath around 5pm and told my other half to call the hospital at 6pm and tell them we were on our way as the surges were so close together at this point that I couldn't time them. The hospital, knowing it was my first baby, said to wait another hour. I said I wasn't waiting and tried to rush my other half to leave.

The trip to the hospital felt like an eternity as it was so bumpy.

When I got to triage around 7pm it turned out I was fully dilated and my body needed to push. We just had enough time to fill the pool and my little boy, Dylan was born at 8:04pm on December 30th. I'm now expecting my second and hoping for another positive story soon.

Louise and baby Dylan

The birth of Jenson

I found out about Claire and The Nurture Nest during my second pregnancy when I was searching HYPNOBIRTH podcasts and I loved them! I started from the beginning and went back on episodes I wanted reassuring on, like induction, and liked listening to all the positive birth stories.

For my second birth I really wanted a water birth, but I was open minded and knew that things can change and I had accepted that it may not be just like my first birth.

This time round I was made aware of strep B and my hospital was doing trials so I opted to do the swab test at 36 weeks and found I was positive so I knew I would need antibiotics whilst in labour.

17 days before my "due date" I was sorting out my kitchen and my Mum was helping me de frost the freezer and clean the oven, I was sorting out and re organising my cupboards and that night my waters broke about 11pm, so I rang the hospital and they said as I'm strep B positive they would like to see me, so I rang my Mum to come and collect Holly and our dog Jeeves and headed for the hospital.

We discussed that as my waters had broken and I'm strep B positive it's advised to have the baby within 24 hours due to infections. I was offered an induction there and then but I said I would like to try and start on my own, and I said let's give it 12 hours and so an appointment to be induced was made for 2pm the next day. In the back of my mind I was really dreading the induction, but I knew I needed to accept the change of direction. Luckily at my hospital the monitors are wireless so a water birth was still possible and I would be able to move, my fear was being strapped to a bed!

We went home and I managed to get some sleep and chill in the morning listening and relaxing to my music and tracks. No labour signs came so we went to hospital and we were given a birthing room with pool, which I was so excited about. I listened to my tracks and chill music whilst we waited for the antibiotics for the strep B to start.

At 5:35pm the antibiotics started and then after about 30 minutes the hormone drip started at a low amount, nothing really happened for the first hour so I sent Kyle home to get some tea. Then mild period pains started and I thought oooh it's happening! Then they started to get more intense but it didn't feel all of a sudden just a good steady pace, but things were moving! I had seen somewhere that using a comb on the palms of your hand and squeezing when having a contraction helps so when they started to get a little more intense I grabbed the beard comb and never let it go until he was born, it was the best thing and highly recommend this little trick.

The midwife didn't want to examine me too much due to risk of infections so we had set a time at 11:30pm to see how I was going, However at about 11pm I said I feel like I need to push! So the pool was ready and in I got, and began pushing. I had Kyle on one side, the student midwife on the other and the main midwife focusing on me letting me breathe through and encouraging me which I really appreciated, she let me feel the head and then after a final push/ breath, I pulled Jenson up and he was so calm and chilled, Kyle was offered to cut the cord but didn't fancy it so I did, it was amazing and I felt that Kyle was really involved in the birth and supported me perfectly.

After getting out of the pool I birthed the placenta which was very quick and painless, I didn't expect it to be. I was then examined to see if I had any tearing and I was amazed to find out nothing! I was so pleased I managed to breathe Jenson out with no pain relief, no tearing, I did it with the support of Kyle, the midwives and just holding my mega beard comb.

Thank you Claire for your amazing podcast it really helped me through my pregnancy and birth and I've recommended you to so many people!

Deborah and baby Jenson

VBAC

The birth of Matilda

My second daughter's birth was incredibly different to her sisters. 2 years and 1 month after my first labour ended in an unplanned caesarean, I wanted so desperately to have a VBAC (vaginal birth after caesarean). Being that I was a "c-section Mum" I was put into a high-risk category. Through many meetings and conversations with Claire, my husband and I decided we absolutely knew a VBAC was something me and the baby could achieve. I wanted to give birth in hospital because of the slight increase in risk of my caesarean scar rupturing and agreed to be heavily monitored during this time.

It was the most beautiful birth, with twinkly fairy lights in the room and my hypnobirthing music playing, assisted by wonderful midwives who were also hypnobirthing trained and supportive.

My waters were artificially broken for me, so I did need a little help with pain relief, and Matilda ended up being a forcep delivery. The support from the hospital for my VBAC and my conversations over the phone with Claire during my labour to give me the little bit of extra hypnobirthing support I needed made Matilda's birth a really amazing experience for everyone involved. I was so proud that we managed to achieve the VBAC birth I wanted.

Marie and baby Matilda

The birth of Raife

Raife is my third birth. My first daughter was an unplanned c-section, my second daughter was a VBAC induction (with the help of forceps), so this time, I wanted to birth with as little interference to me and the baby as possible and birth at home.

Since the birth of my second daughter, we had come mostly through COVID, there was still the odd guideline in place (midwives wearing masks etc.), but mostly life was pretty much back to our new normal. We decided it was time to have a complete refresher full hypnobirthing Course with the wonderful Claire - The Nurture Nest, and this made my husband and I realise we had so much to process from the previous two births, which we talked through. We both agreed that for our third baby, we wanted to be at home, with the support of midwives. My husband did a lot of reading and research in being the best birth partner he could be for us, and one thing stuck out, which was a "safe word", if things got too much, we needed to move to the next plan.

Being that I was a previous VBAC I still had to be consultant led. Which meant I needed to sign lots of paperwork to have an HBAC, but I was certain this was the right thing for me and my baby.

For this birth, I refused any sweeps as they did not help me previously, this time my body went into spontaneous labour completely by itself. I had a mucus plug show the day before, and woke very early in the morning around 4am with surges, which I knew were the real thing. When my husband woke at 6am I told him he should take our daughters who were 2 and 4 to their grandparents, so I knew that I did not need to worry about them, and we could carry on with our day as normally as possible with the hopes that labour would progress without chasing it.

Once he had pulled back onto our driveway after dropping the girls, my surges became consistent and stronger. I pottered around the kitchen, folded some washing, and ate a punnet of grapes, until it got too uncomfortable to continue to do small things.

We then decided to put on a funny film, and I used a comb in my hand to help me through the surges, I had a chat on the phone from my hypnobirthing teacher Claire, who gave me some wise, calming words after which, things became more intense and I felt I needed to get into my birthing zone. I put a calming background on the TV, which was something from YouTube, a hypnobirthing music playlist, a lavender candle, low lighting and curtains closed, it felt like a very safe space. At this point the surges felt very strong and frequent. My husband called the birth unit to inform a midwife, who would come and visit to see how we were getting on in the next couple of hours. It was so peaceful and calm, and my husband was very present with me. I needed his focus on me and nowhere else, which stayed that way for the entire birth.

Within around 40 minutes, the midwife arrived, I had not met her before, she slipped into the room and settled on a sofa to observe me for some time. She asked if she could do an internal examination to determine whether I was in active labour or not. Due to the intensity of the surges I wanted to know if I was in active labour (past 4cm dilated). My husband checked with me that this is what I really wanted to ensure I was not feeling pressured into it, but I did want it. In that snapshot of time, I was 4cm dilated, in active labour, so the midwife was staying. There was a sense of relief at this point, because it had felt quite intense and I wanted to have some light relief from the gas and air. I held off for another hour or so before asking for the gas and air as I knew I could cope. I tried many different positions to get comfortable, all fours, leaning over the sofa, my husband massaging my lower back, I then had some gas and air which was a huge relief and felt like I was able to rest a little more between surges to keep some energy. As a previous C-section, it was agreed I would have intermittent fetal heart rate monitoring, so every 20 minutes or so, she checked his heart rate with a portable doppler, and he was unphased and consistent all through the birth. A second midwife arrived and I remember hearing them whisper chatting whilst I was leaning on my husband and riding through the surges. The shape of my bump changed after a few hours, and it felt as if the baby was close, my waters were still intact. The midwives had set up a little area for the baby once he was here in the corner of the room. Very quickly on all fours, I felt the need to push, which was not the baby, but instead a balloon of waters, which came out of me but did not burst. This was the strangest sensation, the waters stayed intact and were dangling, this made me feel very uncomfortable.

The midwives then received a phone call from the birth unit at the hospital, informing them their shift was coming to an end and homebirths were being cancelled for the evening due to staff shortages. They both informed me it was their duty to stay with me, but they had been on a long shift and in the hospital there were fresh midwives should I choose to go in. I declined.

I continued to labour at home for another hour or so, but the interruption stalled me somewhat. The midwives wanted to check I did not have any meconium in my waters, so asked to burst them, which I agreed to, and they were clear, so no meconium, which meant I did not medically need to transfer into hospital, I could continue to labour at home. It was evening by this time and I was getting very tired. There was a suggestion that the baby had a hand by his face, which was stopping him from coming down, but at this point having a walk around was not possible. The midwives decided to call an ambulance "just in case" we needed to transfer in. A mix of the pressure of knowing the midwives wanted to go into the hospital, the ambulance waiting outside and my sheer exhaustion; I used our safe word, my husband looked me dead in the eye and asked me if that was really what I wanted, I confirmed it was.

We took a short 7 minute ambulance ride to the hospital, which was incredibly bumpy and I felt on the entire journey that I needed to push, I was being told not to push, over and over again.

We arrived at the hospital, and I got immediately put in a room, my husband lifted me onto the bed and I instinctively was on all fours, holding on to handles at the top of the bed. Very quickly I had more gas and air, and within 15 minutes at 8:15pm our little boy was handed under my leg, both of us getting caught up in his nuchal cord and I was sitting up on my knees holding him, with the feeling of sheer relief. "All you needed was a little jiggle in an ambulance" the midwife who had stayed with me from home said. I had to have a couple of stitches, which I was numbed for and recovered very quickly from.

Although it was not the HBAC I wanted, 95% of his birth was at home. I managed to come home quickly the next morning and by 2pm in the afternoon his sisters were back at home and we were a family of 5 in that wonderful baby bubble that no words can truly describe.

Marie and baby Raife

The birth of Harry

The first time I gave birth was to my daughter in January 2021, during lockdown. I was induced at 39 weeks due to reduced movements. Long story short, it took 4 days, I had to be alone and it was quite traumatic. Eventually Millie came via unplanned c section, following 3 hours of pushing and failed forceps. Ben (my partner) then had to leave us after an hour of his daughter being born. It was awful and to this day I believe our experience has a lot to answer for as to why Millie (my daughter) was a very difficult baby.

When I fell pregnant again in August 2022 I soon started worrying about how I was going to have to give birth again. I knew I had two options, elective c-section or a VBAC (vaginal birth after caesarean) each of which comes with its' own advantages and disadvantage.

Through my pregnancy I focused on hypnobirthing (I honestly can't recommend it enough). Hypnobirthing changed the way I perceived my body and its' ability to grow and birth a tiny human. I practiced daily and it gave me something to focus on and made me feel in control. I was also extremely lucky to have an incredible midwife who supported me and empowered me to make decisions for myself using tools and facts.

Towards the end of my pregnancy I was excited to give birth. As part of my birth preferences I had stated that I would not be induced and unless I went into spontaneous labour by 41 weeks I would have an elective c-section. I agreed to start sweeps from 38 weeks, I had 2 in total. Alongside I also had some acupuncture to help my body go into spontaneous labour. In hindsight I think this was the game changer.

I had been having lots of Braxton Hicks for about 2 weeks and feel that I was probably in early labour for a long time. On the 7th May, I was up at 4am and felt the sensations were changing. I carried on with my day as normal and went to a Coronation picnic with my family. While we were there I continued to have very irregular period type pains. I felt exhausted and we left to go home at around 3pm.

We got home and I had a shower, still having contractions but they were irregular and far apart. By 5pm they were every 10mins. My daughter hadn't napped that day and was having tantrums and climbing all over me. It was very intense. Ben tried to keep her out the way but I feel she just knew something was going on. As Ben was giving her dinner and putting her to bed things kept ramping up. I was texting a couple of friends and telling them how I wish I'd just gone for a c-section again and I couldn't do this for hours as I was already exhausted.

I showered and relaxed once home. At 6.12pm I rung the midwife to let her know my contractions were about 10 minutes apart and asked for advice as I felt they were becoming quite intense. As I was on the phone I had another contraction and she actually informed me it had only been 3 minutes since the last one and I should be making my way in. Ben was still trying to settle Millie to bed. I then rung Ben's Mum to come for childcare. As she arrived my contractions were coming in fast and we left for the hospital. The car journey was so intense, I felt every bump and tried to breathe through the pain but as things were moving so fast I did panic a bit and actually tried to get out of the car. I used my hypnobirthing breathing and knowledge to regain control. My partner also helped me stay calm and reminded me that this was normal and my body was just preparing.

As we got to the hospital Ben checked the time, 6.59pm, he had 30 minutes to get back to the car and put it in the proper car park before he would get fined. As we got to triage they asked me for a urine sample, as I got into the toilet my waters broke and I didn't feel like I was able to move off the toilet. The midwives quickly rushed me into the nearest delivery room and asked if they could check how dilated I was. In order to do this they needed me to get onto the bed but I found this very difficult and just wanted to stay upright and crouched down. But due to my previous c section they wanted to monitor baby throughout labour, I agreed to this as I was also worried about the small risk of scar rupture.

As I got onto the bed my body started to push on its own. I told them there was no need to check me as I was 10cm and he was coming but I don't think they believed me as everything was happening so quickly.

They were unable to monitor baby properly so they had to use an attachment that they place on baby's head. I had read about them and understood the risks and consented to this. Although on my birth preferences I had said that I didn't want this device I felt this was important at the time as from the doppler reading baby's heart rate was dipping and we needed to know if he was okay. His heart rate was not going above 100 and my section scar was beginning to hurt. This was a concern so they pressed the emergency button. So many people flooded the room and were ready to intervene. I focused and listened to the midwives and Ben, I pushed with everything I had and baby's head was out. 1 more push later and at 7.29pm baby boy was born, despite this situation, due to hypnobirthing I managed to stay centered and calm.

It was the most incredible feeling and the absolute flood of love took over me. He was placed straight onto my chest and I felt like I'd just won the most precious gift in the world. We managed to do delayed cord clamping and had that golden hour. I had to ask Ben to take a picture of his face to show me as he was so close to my face I couldn't see him properly. He was absolutely beautiful.

The third stage of labour wasn't so easy. I found birthing the placenta quite annoying and painful, I just wanted to enjoy my baby. I also had to have some stitching which was also very uncomfortable. I had missed my chance for pain relief but had gas and air through the repairs luckily.

This experience has been so different to my first birth and I am grateful for my positive birth, it has been so healing. I am so proud of what my body achieved and would do it a million times over. Although birth is intense and unpredictable, thanks to hypnobirthing and great antenatal support I felt in control and prepared. I trusted my body and felt like an absolute goddess that I'd manage to push out a perfect human so well.

The real deal breaker here was that I was armed with information and I wasn't afraid to voice my preferences. I also had an incredibly supportive partner who did hypnobirthing with me and took his role seriously. VBACs are 75% successful and risks are very small if labour is spontaneous. Recovery is quicker. It was a no brainer for me.

I'm so lucky it all went well and we got our little Harry to show for it

Margot and baby Harry

INDEX

AMNIOTIC FLUID – a clear, slightly yellowish liquid that surrounds the unborn baby (fetus) during pregnancy.

APGAR – a quick way for health professionals to evaluate the health of newborns at 1 and 5 minutes after birth.

BACK TO BACK – when the back of a baby's head and spine is against the mother's spine during pregnancy.

BLOODY SHOW – common in late pregnancy when a small amount of blood and mucus is released from the vagina. Also known as: mucus plug.

BRAIN – a technique for decision making during pregnancy and birth. Stands for BENEFITS, RISKS, ALTERNATIVES, INSTINCT and NOTHING.

BRAXTON HICKS – random contractions and relaxation of the uterine muscle. Can also be known as false labour or practice labour.

BREAST CRAWL – the instinctive movement of a newborn toward the nipple of its mother for the purpose of latching on to initiate breastfeeding.

BREECH – when the baby is positioned head up and either feet, bottom or knee first during pregnancy.

BUSCOPAN – a medication to relieve stomach cramps.

CANNULA – a small tube that has been placed into a vein in your arm or your hand to deliver intravenous therapy.

CLARY SAGE – an essential oil thought to help induce contractions of the uterus. Should only be used from 37 weeks. Always consult a doctor before using.

COLOSTRUM – the first form of breastmilk that is released after giving birth. It is nutrient-dense and high in antibodies.

CORD PROLAPSE – the descent of the umbilical cord through the cervix alongside or past the presenting part in the presence of ruptured membranes.

CTG – Cardiotocography is a technique used to monitor the fetal heartbeat and uterine contractions during pregnancy and labour.

DELAYED CORD CLAMPING – when extra time is given before clamping the umbilical cord, allowing for extra blood flow from the placenta to the baby after birth.

DIAMORPHONE – an opioid pain relief medicine.

DOPPLER – a device that uses sound waves to detect movement – such as that of a heartbeat.

DOULA – a person who supports women and birthing people through labour and birth and/or after the baby is born.

DOWN BREATHING – a breathing technique for use during the second stage of labour.

ECV – external cephalic version. A procedure to try and turn a baby from a breech position into a head-down position.

EJECTION REFLEX – when the body expels a baby involuntarily, without forced pushing.

EPIDURAL – an injection into your back to stop you feeling pain in part of your body.

EPISIOTOMY – a cut made by a healthcare professional into the perineum to make more space for a baby to be born. See also: perineum

GBS – Group B Strep. A common bacteria that can live in the vagina.

GOLDEN HOUR – the first hour after birth when a mother has uninterrupted skin-to-skin with the newborn. A critical time for a newborn.

INDUCTION – a process that prompts the uterus to contract during pregnancy before labour begins on its own.

IUI – a type of fertility treatment.

MASTITIS – an inflammation of breast tissue that sometimes involves an infection.

MECONIUM – a newborn's first poo. This sticky, thick, dark green poo is made up of cells, protein, fats, and intestinal secretions, like bile.

MEMBRANE - layers of tissue called the amniotic sac that hold the fluid that surrounds the baby in the womb.

MILES CIRCUIT – a series of positions that help to move your baby into a favourable position.

MOXIBUSTION – a traditional Chinese medicine therapy where dried mugwort leaves are burnt on particular points on the body.

OXYTOCIN – a hormone. Its main function is to facilitate childbirth.

PERINEUM – tiny patch of skin between the vagina and the anus.

PETHIDINE – an opioid pain relief medicine.

PROPESS TAMPON – a form of induction. Looks like a small tampon that is inserted into the cervix in order to encourage dilation.

PROSTAGLANDINS – a hormone. Sometimes used as part of the induction process to soften and ripen the cervix.

RHESUS NEGATIVE – a blood type.

RING OF FIRE – the circle your baby's head makes as it pushes on and stretches the vaginal opening. Can cause a burning/stinging sensation.

SKIN TO SKIN – when the baby is laid directly on their mother's chest straight after childbirth. Very beneficial for both mother and baby.

SURGE – another name for a contraction during labour.

SWEEP – technically a form of the induction process. A process of trying to encourage labour to start.

SYNTOCINON – a synthetic version of the hormone oxytocin. Used as part of the induction process.

TENS MACHINE – transcutaneous electrical nerve stimulator. A small, battery-operated device that uses electrical impulses to help reduce pain signals going to the spinal cord and brain.

TRANSITION – a stage of labour that occurs between the first and second stage when the baby's head passes through the cervix and into the vagina.

TRANSVERSE – when a baby is lying sideways across your tummy rather than in a head-down position.

UP BREATHING – a breathing technique to use during the first stage of labour.

VBAC – vaginal birth after caesarean. Also HBAC – home birth after caesarean.

VBB – vaginal breech birth.

VERNIX – a white, sticky substance that covers your baby's skin while in the womb. It acts as a natural moisturiser that helps protect the newborn against infection in the first few days.

For more information on hypnobirthing and to see the courses and services Claire offers, visit **www.thenurturenest.co.uk**.

For further support during your pregnancy follow Claire on Instagram @the_nurture_nest and have a listen to the number 1 podcast, The Hypnobirthing Podcast. Available on all the main podcast platforms.